THE GIFT

of A STOLEN

YOUTH

TIHANA BABIC

First published in Australia by Aurora House
www.aurorahouse.com.au

This edition published 2021
Copyright © Tihana Babic 2021

Cover design: Donika Mishineva
www.artofdonika.com
Typesetting and e-book design: Amit Dey

ISBN number: 978-1-922403-88-9 (paperback)

NATIONAL LIBRARY OF AUSTRALIA
A catalogue record for this book is available from the National Library of Australia

Distributed by: Ingram Content: www.ingramcontent.com
Australia: phone +613 9765 4800 |
email lsiaustralia@ingramcontent.com
Milton Keynes UK: phone +44 (0)845 121 4567 |
email enquiries@ingramcontent.com
La Vergne, TN USA: phone +1 800 509 4156 |
email inquiry@lightningsource.com

We can complain because rose bushes have thorns or rejoice because thorn bushes have roses.

—Alphonse Carr

To my parents:
thank you for being the reason I smile.

Acknowledgements

◇

I want to dedicate this book to my two guardian angels – my parents: my mother, Mirela, and my father, Zvonimir. If it were not for them, I never would have made it this far. With their love, compassion, watchfulness, care and immense understanding, they were and still are my rocks. Their support helped me a great deal, and not just that, it made me want to succeed. Having backup makes a great difference. It's like having a safety net behind you 24/7. In my case, there were two of them, so it was nearly impossible to fall. This is all metaphorical, of course, but really what they did for me cannot be summed up in words. I know that it's a parent's duty to support their child, but this went way beyond caring and supporting. Their endless love, compassion and helping hands deserve separate thanks.

To my mother – a big, big, immense thank you. I cannot count all the times you helped me, were there for me and listened when I needed someone to hear me out. Not just listened, but also understood my fears without judgement or blame. My unreasonable thoughts and views were always reviewed, not disregarded or made to seem unimportant. There were so many times when I needed, and still need, guidance. You firmly stood by me and always made me feel better about myself. Even when the prognosis wasn't so good, you brushed your own fears aside and continued reassuring me not to give up. You always encouraged me to keep on fighting and give it my best. It will never be forgotten. You are my force! Thank you.

To my father – a huge thank you, a million times over. You were always there for me, providing help, care and understanding, even when I didn't entirely deserve it. Countless times my behaviour towards you was rude, inappropriate and inadequate. I blamed you for everything that happened, and you took that blame willingly, without resistance. My behaviour was disrespectful, mean and unnecessary. From the bottom of my heart, I regret it and apologise to you. Thank you for tolerating that behaviour, and despite it all, continuing to give me endless love and support. You were that person who pushed me beyond my boundaries. You never ceased to believe in me, always reassuring me that I could achieve whatever I wanted. There are no boundaries; I just have to believe to make things happen. The best way to put it in words, you are the engine that powers me and keeps me going. Thank you.

To both my parents: thank you for being the reason I smile!

I also want to thank all the people who helped me through my journey, which was packed with ups and downs. It was a bad experience and all of these people contributed to make it better.

First and foremost, a big thank you to all the doctors and nurses who treated me. They helped me through my struggles and gave me the reassurance that I could carry on.

Well, some of them did, while most of them not so much. I am badmouthing them throughout my book; I am completely aware of that. But every single thing noted did indeed happen. I didn't make up or imagine anything. Unfortunately, my not-so-good pathway was worsened by their deeds, and that hurt. It still does. I'm now realising that I've lost my trust in them. All the grief and sorrow their actions caused has engraved a very deep, negative feeling in me towards any doctor.

Secondly, my physiotherapists, occupational therapists and speech therapists deserve a great big thank you for tolerating me when I wasn't in a good mood and when the sessions were mixed with tears. Their main goal was to train me for an independent and valuable life despite my disabilities. I must single out two people with whom I've created a special bond and who I respect a great deal. The first person is my physiotherapist, Zhao. He is truly a miracle worker – so much compassion, understanding, and above all, knowledge. I have worked with countless physio-therapists, but none of them comes close to him. His immense knowledge speaks volumes. Your work will never be forgotten! The second person is my speech therapist, Carolin. She helped me, understood me, believed in me and encouraged me as I fought my battles. She is still trying and succeeding in diminish-ing the effects this misery brought me. A big thankyou for all your help and belief in me.

Thirdly, to all the people who supported me – my companions and support people, you not only upgraded my social life, but also let light into the darkness that was slowly consuming me. Thank you! I need to single out one person in particular because she's not just a support person, she's a friend and confidante. Too many times she stepped out of the provider-client relationship and showed genuine care, love and support. She even moved into the personal side of my life and helped. Thank you, Trudi for being a true friend.

Finally, I want to thank every organisation that provided financial help and other benefits. There were many times when I received a wide variety of help, either in the form of therapy or various aids. I thank Australia for everything I received and for everything I am still receiving. Without the hard work of so many people, none of this would be possible. I am so grateful.

Contents

◇

Prologue

*To live is to suffer. To survive is to find some meaning
in the suffering.*

~Friedrich Nietzsche

Everyone suffers. You are not alone. It is common for people
to hide their aches and pains to the point that they get lost
in their own lies and hiding games. Personally, I cannot understand this. Perhaps they are too embarrassed to address their problems. Maybe they want to paint the picture of an idyllic family
with no worries or troubles. I have met several people who want
to show off their perfect life. They look you in the eye and lie.
What astonishes me is that they are convinced their bubble will
never burst. Don't they know their lies will be revealed in time?
Can't they see that they are only conning themselves? Like the
Croatian proverb says, 'The Earth made a pledge to Heaven that
all its secrets shall be revealed'.

Suffering is part of life. The only difference is that some people suffer more than others. Sadly, that is the way it is. Sometimes though, it seems that some people are destined to suffer

throughout their lifetimes, while others experience little or none. *Is the scale out of order?* I guess our only consolation is to bear in mind that by endurance we conquer.

In writing this book and sharing my misfortune with others, I am liberating myself from secrets buried deep inside. By secrets I mean events that scarred my life. I wish to share them with you and show that there is a way to overcome these strokes of bad luck successfully. It is not easy, but my story can surely testify that it is possible. My battle gave me a firsthand view of life's challenges and horrifying changes. Nevertheless, a great battle in my life has been won, not once, but twice. Therefore, hope exists. You can fight any misery and give it your best to succeed. I am not saying every illness or adversity can be overcome. Trust me, beating an illness is not a piece of cake. It cannot be overcome effortlessly. Every illness takes its toll. Fighting for your health is stressful, draining, and physically and mentally painful. All I am saying is that facing the battle with a positive approach helps. Positive thinking combined with positive action results in success. *Worked for me twice!*

This is not bragging. My share of suffering and worrying was more than enough. Sometimes I think I did not just get a cross to bear but a whole crucifixion as well. Nonetheless, a person should be as positive as they can be. I passionately believe my positive approach towards life and willingness to fight kept me – and is keeping me – alive. The attitude you have towards life and living determines your path!

This book is packed with tips and advice on maintaining health – everything I have tried that was effective. I hope my story will help someone. If I can reassure someone else about their situation, or alleviate another's suffering, then this was not in vain.

'Although the world is full of suffering, it is also full of the overcoming of it.'[1]

---

[1] Helen Keller, American author.

1

La Vita è Bella

◇

Life is full of beauty. Notice it.

~Ashley Smith

ere is an introduction to my story and my views on certain aspects of life. My beliefs and assurances helped me through my journey. Some of my principles may be too strict, but most of them have served me well. In some things – exercise and other physical activities, especially – strictness and abidance are necessary to vanquish a problem.

Have you seen the movie *La Vita è Bella* with Roberto Benigni in the main role? It is a beautiful, tear-jerking movie, and it shows life's true colours. It vividly paints a picture of life's cruellest moments. A viewer can see the struggle of a father who creates a game out of a horrific situation in order to make things less painful for his son. I watched it once and doubt it I will have the strength to watch it again. As the title indicates, even in its darkest hours, life is beautiful and worth living.

That's my philosophy. I believe life can be cruel and ugly, but it can also be thrilling and wonderful. In my opinion, it is the wonderful moments that give us the courage and strength to get through tough times. One's memories are the secret strength. My life, so far, has been throwing me in all directions, a rollercoaster ride gone terribly wrong. Thankfully, my will and strength helped me survive. Not only that, there were lots of well wishers who gave me much needed 'pats on the back'.

My health problems started in 1999. I was a sixteen-year-old high-school student. As time progressed, my illness, or should I say the symptoms of my illness, worsened. Finally, in March 2003, I was diagnosed with a malignant brain tumour – cancer. I was eighteen. In 2009, the cancer returned. At that stage I was twenty-four. My adolescence and youth were flushed down the toilet.

Once I got through the pain and suffering my first tumour brought, I began resetting and refreshing my mind, body and soul. I enjoyed six years of semi-normal life where I attended university and formed a path to a new future. Sadly, my new plan was shattered into little pieces – particles to be precise – by the recurrence. It was a horrible time in my life that blemished and stigmatised my existence. Thankfully, I have been able to overcome certain things, but the aftermath and its impact linger on. Fighting them day in and day out is something I cannot dismiss or make disappear. Everything that happened severely damaged my life, but my only option was – and is – to keep on battling with a positive attitude.

My experiences taught me an important lesson – the immense value of good health. They say that the greatest wealth in life is health. Before my distressing event, I took my good health for granted. It never occurred to me that health was something to be nourished and maintained. It is funny how we humans treat it. Yesterday, my life was in jeopardy. I didn't know whether I would live or die. Today, when everything is okay, I treat my health with the same contempt I did before I got sick. As soon as everything is alright, we revert to an ignorant state where good health is assumed and not prioritised. It is sometimes nice to be ignorant and follow your urges. But sometimes the price for doing so is sky high. I think that people, myself included, should seriously start shifting their priorities, and comprehend that a person who has their health has everything.

Another thing I learnt is that I do not like quitting. The words 'giving up' do not exist for me. Maybe that belief helped me get over my misfortune. Everyone can quit; it is so easy. But fighting and giving it all you've got makes all the difference. If you quit, you are depriving yourself of the possibility of ever succeeding. You might fail or succeed, but you will never know if you quit. Quitting is fine if you're dead. But I believe that if you are breathing, you are not entitled to quit. This is not a religious statement. Nonetheless, I believe in fighting; I believe in activity, because by doing that the only outcome can be success. In my opinion, fighting is a much better option. At least you will have the satisfaction of knowing you tried.

If someone were to ask me 'How did you do it?' or 'What made you go ahead and fight?', my answer would not be satisfying. It would be vague. Maybe it was my internal motivation about not quitting or not allowing myself to stay in that bad condition. Adding to all that, I'm a perfectionist: a self-oriented one who adheres to perfection in order to avoid failure. Generally, perfectionism is considered a hindrance, but it helped me a lot along my path. It made me want to try again when things failed.

There is one more thing that has had an impact – anger. At first, I did not give this much thought, but now I am positive that anger plays a big role in my journey. It is not the kind of anger with lots of bitterness and rage involved, although these feelings are not strangers! It's more like a fuelling anger that doesn't let me quit. Always pushing me forward, encouraging me to say, 'I won't let you beat me', or 'I'm not going down without a fight!' Ultimately, the past cannot be changed but the future can. If I want to enjoy the future, I must fight. After all, not everything in my health war was always so black: there were fifty shades of black, some grey and even a bit of white.

My goal in saying all this is not to give a lecture on how to live life or be a Miss Know-It-All, bragging about how I survived. Rather, I am explaining how I see quitting and giving up.

This goes for everyone: people do not know what their future will be like, but despite that, they strive for a good life. If we knew what would happen in the future, life would be easy. But there'd be no thrill, no excitement. Wouldn't it be kind of dull? Would knowing what will happen next take the buzz out of life? If you knew the future, your every move would be spent eliminating bad things from happening. Daily, your main struggle would be enjoying the good in your life and maintaining harmony. Where is the joy, satisfaction, happiness, or fulfilment in doing that? Maybe some people would like to live that way, but I would not. Disregarding everything that happened in my life, it is kind of interesting not knowing what will happen next.

It comes down to two paths – fight to your last breath or stop fighting and quit. But know that quitting is a path where there is no turning back. Once you quit, you give up all possibilities for a better outcome. There is absolutely nothing to anticipate other than death. It is entirely up to you!

'The only thing we know about the future is that it will be different.'[2]

---

[2] Peter Drucker, businessman.

2

Childhood Memories

◇

*The best and most beautiful things in the world cannot be
seen or even heard but must be felt with the heart.*

~Helen Keller

This chapter explains my life in Croatia, from the moment
I was born in the summer of 1984, to my first departure
for Australia in summer 1988 and onwards. My intention is to
introduce my life prior to the first cancer.

Life was easygoing until 3 March 2003. My childhood and
upbringing were, in a word, beautiful. I was born in 1984 in
Osijek, Croatia and lived there with my parents – Mirela and
Zvonimir – and my grandparents – Miroslava and Ljubomir.
Osijek is located on the left bank of the River Drava, in east-
ern Croatia. It is the largest city in a region called Slavonia. Its
name Osijek comes from the Croatian word *oseka* which means
'ebb tide'. Osijek is a wonderful city, filled with trees and sun, but

above all, history. It traces its roots back to the second century
AD, when its name was Mursa and it was part of the Roman
Empire. The city was almost destroyed by Ottoman conquerors in
the sixteenth century. The Turks rebuilt the city in Ottoman ori-
ental style and called it Ösek. Osijek was part of the Budin Eyalet,
the Ottoman Empire's administrative territorial entity in Cen-
tral Europe and the Balkans. Following the Battle of Mohács in
1526, Osijek was liberated by the Habsburg dynasty. From then
on Osijek was under their reign, which lasted until 28 August
1809 when Osijek became a free royal city – the same day as my
birthday. That was the beginning of a new era in which the city
blossomed even more.

During the First and Second World Wars, Osijek was part
of Kingdom of Yugoslavia, which became the Socialist Federal Republic of Yugoslavia (SFRY) after the Second World
War. On the 25 June 1991, Croatia declared its independence,
which led to the four-year Homeland War[3]. Since then, Osijek
has enjoyed the privileges of an autonomous and independent
city, and has progressed under the secure wing of the Republic
of Croatia.

I really enjoyed living in Osijek. We lived in Retfala, a peaceful and calm suburb in a busy city. *My Osijek!* My mother worked
as a road engineer in Croatia. Later, she was employed in a firm
called Gravia, where she worked as a road designer. My father is

---

[3] Homeland War – civil war of independence that was fought from 1991 to 1995
between Croat forces loyal to the government of Croatia – which had declared independence from the Socialist Federal Republic of Yugoslavia (SFRY) – and the Serb-
controlled Yugoslav People's Army (JNA) and local Serb forces.

a carpenter by trade. He had his own workshop where he made things out of wood – mainly furniture.

Mum, being an only child, was very connected to her parents, Miroslava and Ljubomir. My grandparents were hugely involved in my upbringing. To be honest, for most of my childhood and all my teenage days we lived in their house. I had the misfortune not to meet my dad's father, Ivan, who passed away before my birth. My dad's mother, Ana, passed away when I was seven years old, so I do not remember her. My mum's father, Ljubomir, also passed away early, so my mum's mother, Miroslava, was the only one left of my close family. Not for long though. In general, I have more memories of Mum's parents than Dad's. My wider family or the lack of it is a story of its own, one I will save for another time.

My grandparents, Miroslava and Ljubomir, had a cabin in the hills in a small village called Orahovica. It was a genuinely nice place, filled with greenery, without the rattle of cars and noise. Apparently, I loved visiting. There was a lake so we would often go for a swim. As well as being a holiday resort, my grandfather had a vineyard on the property. Every year, for fun, he would make wine.

When I was four, I started kindergarten where I grew more socialised, although even then, I was not a very sociable person. Mum says that I would call all my friends in the neighbourhood, give them toys to play with and meet their needs, then leave them to play alone.

I loved going out with my parents but very quickly, within five minutes, I would want to go elsewhere. Once they took me to the market. I was so bored that I hid under a table. Everyone was alarmed and the whole market echoed with my name. Later, they found me playing under the table. I did not disobey them frequently, but sometimes I did spit the dummy.

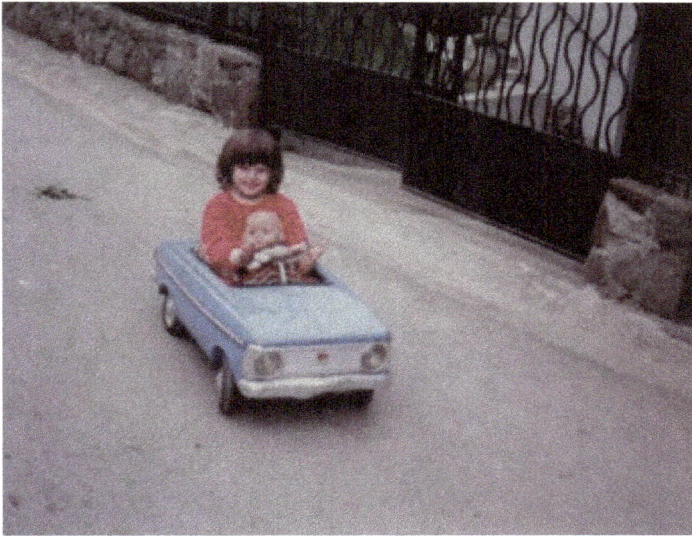

Before Australia

My parents claim that I absolutely adored eating cured or dried meat. In Slavonia, where we lived, people eat a lot of pork, especially cured pork: dried bacon, varieties of sausage, prosciutto… Even now I love it but I can't eat it as much as I used to for health reasons.

My father's dream was to go to Australia. When I was around three years old, he began to make the dream a reality. He spoke to people, applied for a visa, arranged work and so on. In 1987, he booked a flight and was off to live his dream and establish a starter point for Mum and me. His first destination was Sydney where he would find a place to rent. Three months after Dad left, Mum went too. I lived with my grandparents while my parents settled in. I had a nice time with my grandparents. They spoiled me even more, fulfilling all my wishes and giving me all I needed, even when it was unrealistic. Before, I had been my parents' little princess. Now that I was in my grandparents' care, I became their little queen.

Once my parents had set everything up for me to join them (sometime in 1988), the problem was my age. Children under eighteen are not permitted to fly without adult supervision. At that time, my dad's sister Snježana was planning to go to Australia, so she agreed to take me. The flight was scheduled, and the show began. This was the first time I'd been on a plane, but I wasn't scared. I was enthusiastic and happy, looking forward to new adventures, so I have been told. It was a nearly twenty-four-hour flight, but I handled it well. We landed in Sydney and my parents took us to an apartment they had rented.

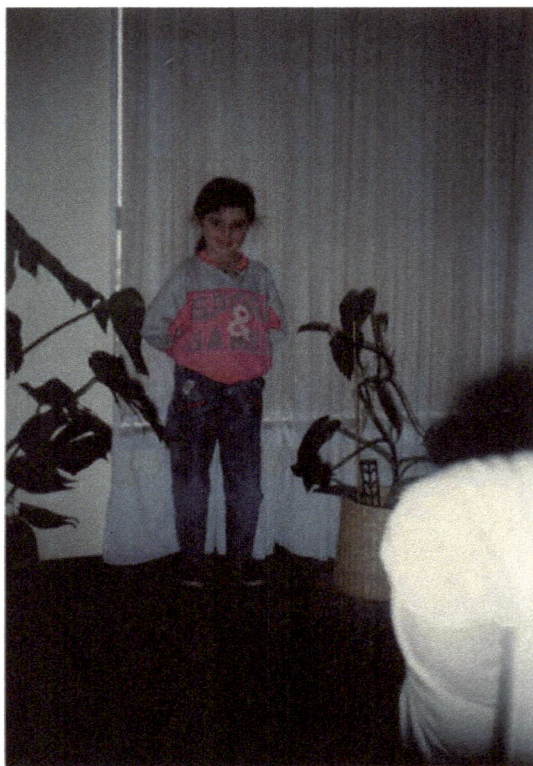

Me in Sydney - 1989

At first, things were very unusual and kind of upside down, with no resemblance to my life in Croatia. And there was the language too! Not knowing how to communicate was daunting. I was safe spending time under my parents' guardian wings, but when I started attending preschool, my troubles began.

Preschool in Australia starts earlier than in Croatia. So, not long after my arrival, I started to go. I remember one episode from preschool that's part funny, part sad. Not knowing very much of the language, I had an issue with a boy. We Croats are very emotional people. When talking and communicating with others we gesticulate and put our hearts into it. Anyway, the boy was playing with a toy for an awfully long time and I wanted to play with it too. He did not want to share. I did not know how to say 'Let's share'. I tried to somehow gesticulate, but he was persistent. I got angry and slapped him. My parents were called in to discuss the unfortunate event. It never happened again but I guess it was not a pleasant experience for Mum and Dad.

At that time, I loved those cars in which a kid could sit in and drive with pedals. I've always been a tomboy. My dad drove all over Sydney to find a car like the one I wanted. I did not have a brand or colour in mind. I just wanted that kind of car. He struggled to find one because kids' cars were a hit in Croatia but had not arrived in Australia yet. Finally, after all the stress, he found a yellow Formula One car. I have been told my enthusiasm for it did not last long. I do not know why; I guess it could be attributed to a child's short attention span.

After about a year, we decided to move to Perth because some business deals came up for Dad. We travelled by plane and sent our stuff by plane too.

We went to a southern suburb of Perth called Hamilton Hill. Things in the Land Down Under slowly began to fall into

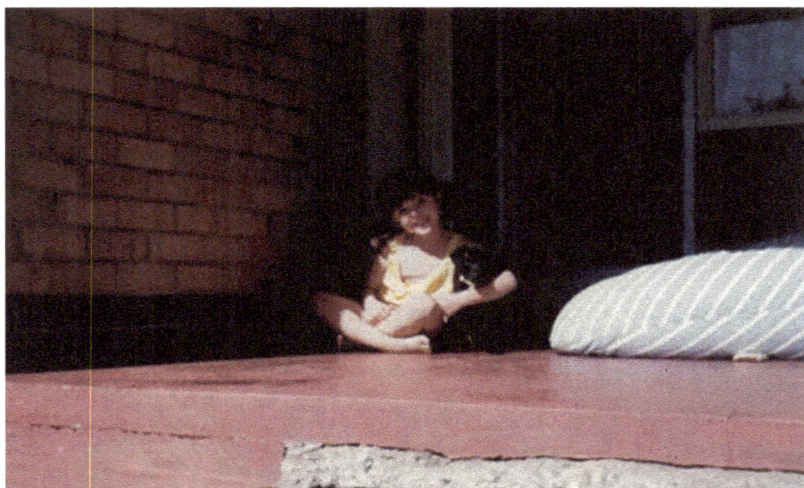

Perth, Western Australia

place, and my adjustment to a new lifestyle was very quick. I learnt English and began to build my future. After preschool, I started primary school where I made many friends. I got seriously involved in playing tennis. I did not have any affinity towards tennis beforehand. My neighbour introduced me to it and I loved it. I was described as promising, and it introduced me to a sporty lifestyle – for a brief period of time.

My Australian adventure was cut short in 1992 when my grandfather, Ljubomir, died. With my grandmother, Miroslava, all alone in a big house, my mum decided to return to Croatia. She would take me with her, and Dad would return later, once he had sorted out all our things and the house we rented in Hamilton Hill. Moving here and there did not bother me much due to my age. Kids adapt quickly. Being eight years old, my view on things was not adult-like. On the one hand, I was sad to leave, mainly because I would miss tennis and did not know if I would continue playing in Croatia or not. On the other hand, I was returning to known things – my house, my grandmother, friends, and Croatian food.

We arrived in Croatia and once again I was starting from the beginning. Mum and I moved into my grandmother's house in Retfala, where we had lived before. Surprisingly, after a couple of months had passed by, I felt like I had never left. My tennis plans sadly came to an end. Hiring tennis courts in Croatia was way more expensive than in Australia. It was hard to let go but I adjusted to no tennis and continued with school and picked different sports. I played a bit of everything – basketball, volleyball, handball. I still played tennis, but it was street tennis. I sometimes wonder 'what if', had I maintained my tennis playing. Maybe my life would have taken another path. I do not know but the 'what if' persists.

Commencing school in Croatia was not easy. Education and knowledge wise, Croatia and Australia are totally different. In Croatia, the first to eighth grades are considered primary school. Another four years are spent in high school, and anything above that is a degree or a trade. My fourth grade in Australian education was equal to the knowledge of second graders in Croatia. So, the second grade was my start. Luckily, I was the same age as the other second graders. This was also because of the differences between the two countries. In Australia, children start school much earlier than in Croatia. My primary school years were blissful. Honestly, I enjoyed school. From primary school to high school to university, I have been successful and found it rewarding, maybe because I was an A-grade student, something close to a nerd. Well, not a complete book worm but close to one.

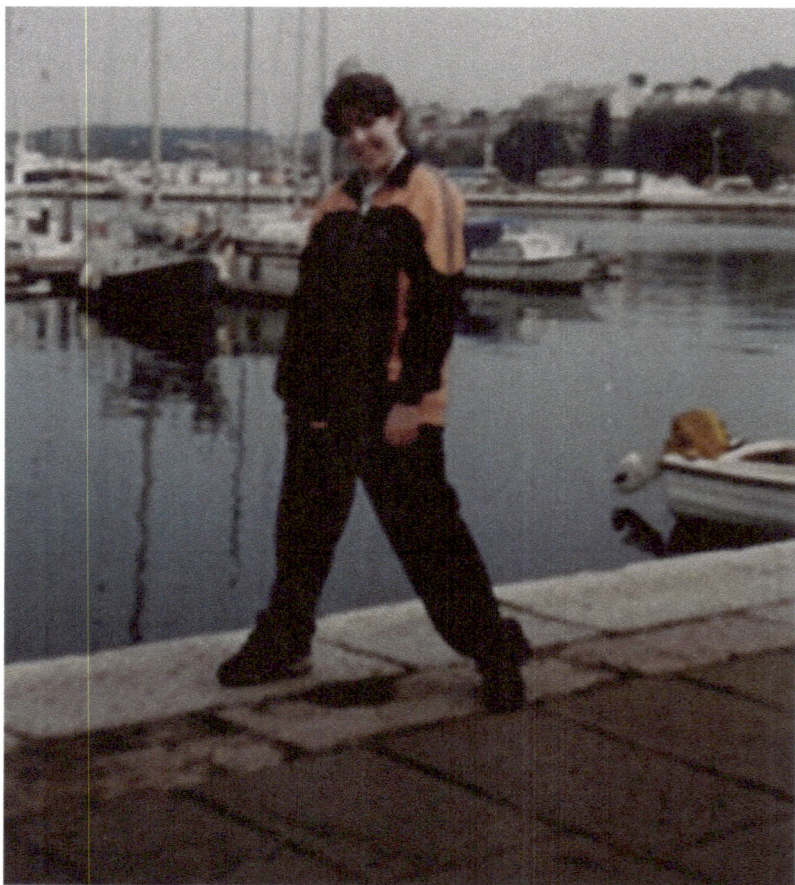

Teenage Years

Apart from school, I did have friends, but I did not like going out every night to discos or anything like that. To be quite truthful, I was not an outgoing person at all. Rather, I was introverted and self-sufficient in everything I did. I loved reading, puzzles, models and TV soaps. I like reading romance novels; I got that from my grandmother, who loved reading romance novels too. I enjoyed learning. Knowledge is always welcome. I particularly like those brainy sentences like 'The great wall in China can be seen from space'. Puzzles and models of cities or buildings interest me, and the more pieces the merrier! I absolutely adore Spanish soap operas; I learnt Spanish from watching them. Now I watch Turkish, Italian and Croatian soap operas.

The start of my teenage years was marked by madness over the Backstreet Boys, an American boyband consisting of five guys – Nick, A.J., Brian, Howie and Kevin. I was obsessed with them. I hoarded all their merchandise: magazines, posters, T-shirts, cups, flags, clothes, CDs, video tapes, DVDs. I had quite the collection. If it were valued, it would have amounted to a big sum of money. But it did not stop there. I transformed my behaviour and appearance according to theirs. I wore wide, baggy clothes; talked American English; had the same hairdo as my favourite Backstreet Boy, Nick Carter, of course; learnt all the dances to their songs; started to use the same words as they used in sentences. It was true craziness, insanity even! Sadly, they did not have concerts in Croatia back then. When eventually they did have a concert, I was unable to go due to the aftermath of my first operation. When they had another concert in Zagreb in 2011, the main issue was the volume. After the recurrence in 2009, I could not handle loudness. A bad headache would occur. Still love the BSBs though!

3

Symptoms

◇

One of the greatest diseases is to be nobody to anybody.

~**Mother Teresa**

In 1999, I finished primary school. I was fifteen years old and enrolled in high school – Grammar School III in Osijek. We call a grammar school a gymnasium in Croatia. It is a high school with a strong emphasis on academic learning. The gymnasium I chose was focused on science and mathematics. I wanted to study aviation or architecture at university one day, hence my choice.

My health problems started in high school. As my illness pro-gressed, or should I say the symptoms of my illness worsened, high school became a problem. I was diagnosed in 2003, but my suspicious symptoms appeared much earlier, four years earlier, to be exact. My symptoms were not considered alarming for the first two years. It all started with strange vision. When I turned my head to the right, my vision was blurred and mixed up. At the time, I did not pay too much attention to this, because it was so infrequent. I never told anyone about this symptom because it was not even considered a symptom or an indicator that something may be wrong. Had someone known about it – my parents or my GP – I would have been referred to an ophthalmologist. As I know now, just by looking through an eye, any growth or irregularity in the brain can be detected. I am not sure to what degree, in terms of measuring size, but some things can be discovered much earlier. Had my tumour been discovered earlier, it would have completely altered the outcome. I am not saying the tumour could have been averted, but the size of it affected the repercussions. A lot of pain, frustration and anger could have been avoided. In the first year of high school that one symptom – occasional blurred vision – dominated. Nothing else was visible. Maybe a headache here and there, but that did not differ from the ones in the past.

Going into my second year of high school, I picked up another symptom, and this one was painful. My stomach started hurting profoundly. The only time the pain would stop is when I lay down. This symptom, along with the first one, and periodic headaches were ongoing for two years. During that time, I started sleeping a lot. It was not like those intentional afternoon naps some people take. It was more like dozing off to a song. Slowly, this became an everyday habit, a thing that came from my body – an inexplicable urge to sleep. This was peculiar because I had never, not once in a blue moon, done anything similar. Now I know that the only time our brain rests and recuperates is during sleep. Everything has an explanation!

All the symptoms started to worry my parents, especially my mum. She never thought much of medicinal tablets. She thought and still thinks that tablets are a quick fix; they give you relief from pain, but they do not eliminate its source. Her beliefs lie more in alternative medicine. At the time she worked for Gravia – a design and construction company – where she heard about an alternative healer from Russia. He was healing people with different illnesses across Croatia. Mum arranged a meeting with him. Supposedly, this guy healed through the eyes. He saw your organs and gave you tablets that he made according to your health problem. The plan was that I should take the tablets he gave me, and after two weeks, I would see improvements with my issues. It did not help me at all. What a total loss of time and money.

Returning to the story, by the end of the third year of high school, the symptoms had become more apparent and occurred more frequently. The weird thing was they could not be linked or attributed to anything. They appeared out of the blue. No prior indications, no nothing. A new symptom occurred between the third and fourth year of high school. We lived in a two-storey house and I would lose my balance coming down the stairs from my room, which was on the first floor. I do not know whether this could be considered a symptom because it was not a drastic loss of balance, more like a wobble, after which I would regain my posture. Thinking about it, it was an indicator that something was not right with my balance; a pointer to the brain or the ears, given that these two control balance.

During the first semester of my fourth year in high school, my absence was very noticeable. I had sick days every week! The pain in my stomach was the worst to deal with. All the symptoms – stomach aches, blurred vision, headaches, falling asleep, loss of balance – were constantly showing up uninvited. A day without at least one of them would not pass. I became a person with an illness, daily anticipating a symptom. It was a horrible time! *But that was just the tip of the iceberg.*

Around October 2002, things were getting more serious, so I started to have all kinds of tests – blood tests, X-rays, a gastroscopy. All the tests were done in Osijek, some in the hospital, some elsewhere, like the GP clinic. Basic tests were done to determine the cause of the symptoms because my doctors thought that all the things were not a big deal. They focused on the stomach pain because it was not normal, I think that was the clearest symptom out of all. In my opinion, they were confused not knowing what symptoms to address.

Looking back, I remember two tests that were awfully bad and painful. I think the clinical staff performed the tests incorrectly, in that they forgot there was a patient – a human being – involved during the procedure.

The first procedure was an X-ray of the upper gastrointestinal tract. Images are produced using a special form of X-ray called fluoroscopy and an orally ingested contrast material such as barium. When the upper GI tract is coated with barium, the radiologist can examine the oesophagus, stomach and duodenum. Doctors use this test to determine why a person's gut is not working properly. It might also help explain why you are losing weight when you do not mean to. A day before the test, I was asked not to eat, drink, or chew gum overnight or on the morning of the test. Your stomach must be empty because food makes it hard to see your GI tract on the X-rays. The X-ray itself was not a problem. The contrast material was! It was chalk in a liquid state. The mix made me vomit. I could barely drink enough for the test. I was sick all day because of it. That one was not painful but disgusting.

The second procedure was a gastroscopy, also known as an upper endoscopy. That one was painful and very unpleasant. They insert a tube (endoscope) into the mouth that travels down the food pipe (oesophagus), then into the stomach and first part of the small intestine to view these areas. The endoscope contains a light and video camera that transmits images to a monitor where they can be seen by a doctor. The bad thing was that I was not anaesthetized at all. In Croatia, they do not do that. Why not? Beats me! Maybe the doctors think that people do not have enough pain in life, so they want more? I have had two gastroscopies, and neither one helped me. They were a complete waste of time and money. If the doctors had looked in the right place, surely it would have given them a clue. Isn't that the job of medicine? Aren't students of medicine thought to unravel the mystery of the unknown?

Nothing came from the tests. All my results were normal, yet my overall state was not.

With time, the symptoms appeared more frequently and with more severity, to the point where I missed school two or three times a week. It was becoming a problem. I remember feeling guilty when I had to call my mum to come and pick me up from school again because the pain was so unbearable. I felt as if I were doing something wrong, as if I purposely wanted to skip school. Not knowing the real cause made me think all kinds of wicked thoughts.

My school reports had not been excellent throughout high school, so I had to pass an extra exam in order to graduate. There was no time to play around. Going to school was an absolute priority and necessity. After all, the plan was for university. Even though I was sometimes in a lot of pain, I got through it.

There was a funny moment among all the bad things happening in that period of my life. At eighteen years old, exactly six months before the revelation of the tumour, I felt on top of the world, like most teens do. Wanting to act smart, I read a book called *The Power of Your Subconscious Mind*. A sentence in it was interesting:

> The splendid secret is the miraculous power of the sub-conscious, which is hidden deep in the mind of every human. If you learn how to recognise and unleash this power of your own intellect, you will bring wealth, pleasure, happiness and health into your life.[4]

I started to comfort myself: maybe I was doing what the book said, without the wealth, pleasure, happiness and health part. *Wishful thinking.*

Anyway, all my professors thought I was bulimic because of my drastic weight loss. I liked being skinny. I had always been chubby before. Now, I felt like Laney coming down the stairs in that teen movie *She's All That.*

Over time, I developed another symptom; I started vomiting profusely. It started in the morning on an empty stomach and lasted until around two or three o'clock in the afternoon. It was like being pregnant. The only catch was that I was lily white. *Maybe it was a miracle conception?* At first the vomiting was once or twice a week. But as time passed, it became very frequent – three or four times a week.

My condition was changeable and very peculiar. Inexplicably, one day I would be sick as hell, and the next two days everything would be okay. Except for the painless symptoms, of course – blurry vision, loss of balance, falling asleep. Those were present 24/7!

By New Year 2002/2003, my condition was not getting any better. Thinking about it now, it was getting worse. Not just worse

---

[4] Dr Joseph Murphy, 1963. *The Power of Your Subconscious Mind* (Englewood Cliffs, New Jersey; Prentice Hall Inc.).

but the worst I'd ever been. My general state was rapidly deteriorating. By the end of February 2003, I could not ignore my health problems. They had become so evident and were affecting my everyday life. At that time, I was not only dealing with the painless symptoms, but the painful ones were present and persistent too. One day, stomach pain, the next day, vomiting, like an unbreakable cycle. A merry-go-round minus the pleasure. Pleasure was lacking, nowhere to be found.

My mother insisted I undergo test after test on top of everything we had tried already, to get to the bottom of this situation. She wanted a thorough examination of my body to understand why all of this was happening. This unpleasant situation had lasted exceedingly long, yet still we could not pinpoint what caused it.

My name became well known in the hospital in Osijek. It was ridiculous. I knew the staff on some wards and we became acquaintances, even friends. Had my appointments been any more frequent, we would have been having tea and making dinner plans. *A pity there were no male nurses.*

When all the tests were over and everything appeared normal, the doctors said I should have an electroencephalography test[5] (EEG) just to make sure everything was fine with my brain. And then, if that was okay, I was to be considered a nut job. They normally did not say it so bluntly, but their faces revealed it. You know that feeling when you can hear words just by looking at someone's face? For now, their official diagnosis was that maybe I was just stressing too much about school. That could have created the symptoms, or maybe I was overly sensitive and took things too

---

[5] Electroencephalography (EEG) is a way of recording the brain's electrical activity by placing electrodes on the scalp.

much to heart. Because they could not give a proper diagnosis, I was a psychological case. Outrageous!

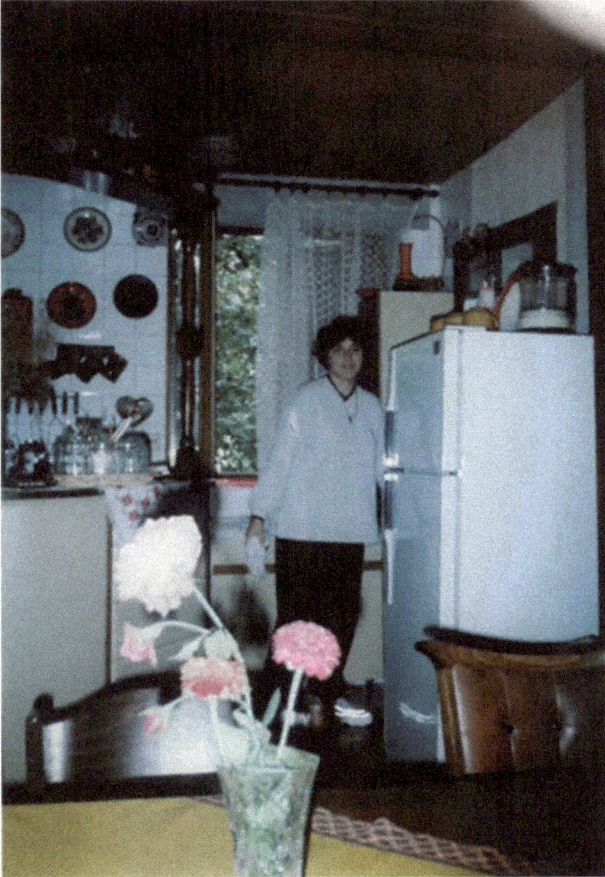

Unravelling fiasco

This fiasco lasted four years. The doctors were playing tennis and I was the ball. In the meantime, my symptoms were not going away; they became more frequent and even more painful. When I think about the doctors' negligence and my mistreatment, my blood boils. My problem was getting bigger by the day, but it was no problem for them. Their lives were not at stake! I do not know how to let go and forget. It still hurts and the pain stays there as if it were yesterday. So persistent. So fixated.

The situation lasted from 1999 to 2003. It could be compared with Dante Alighieri's 'Divine Comedy'. The only difference was that I experienced the nine levels of hell and seven circles of purgatory, with no heaven. Maybe Virgil refused to let me fly off to heaven.

4

Medical Disclosure

◇

What might seem to be a series of unfortunate events may in fact be the first steps of a journey.

~Lemony Snicket

In the last week of February 2003, things started to unravel. The results of my first EEG found irritant dysrhythmic alterations. Though I didn't know what that meant, I instantly saw a red light blinking before my eyes and felt an alarm going off in my head. *Oh no! This is not good. Houston, we have a problem!*

Back then, I didn't know much about problems and disorders of the brain. So, I do not understand why I reacted the way I did. I was not foreseeing anything, nor did I have any indication as to what could have been wrong. The results of the EEG were totally unknown to me. Maybe the word 'irritant' prompted me into thinking something was not right. Basically, at that time I was in ignorant bliss. Ignorance truly was a blessing because knowing the things I know now makes life a living hell.

Nowadays, I cannot even watch children playing in the park without thinking what danger they are putting themselves in. They are doing the exact same things I did when I was a child. In an extremely negative context, 'the knowledge' is just one more 'tattoo' that has been assigned to me – without me asking for it. That tattoo is a constant reminder that I should never forget what happened. Michelle Obama said, 'Every scar that you have is a reminder not just that you got hurt, but that you survived'. Maybe I should look at my scars that way, but it is just so hard when they are still alive and cause so much pain. I would proudly wear the scars if they were not disabling me from doing things or if they did not hurt. All of them would be written on my body, and then I could accurately claim that I do have tattoos. The scars are a constant of what happened, these signs are all over my body and in my memory. They stop me from living my life my way. To somehow calm myself and get myself out of that vicious cycle of thoughts, I called my mother. Some sober thoughts were needed, but as soon as she answered, mischievous words came out.

'Mum, I think I have a brain tumour.'

To this day, I cannot figure out why I said that! Maybe when you are in that negative thought pattern, only bad words come out of your mouth. She did calm me down, console me. But that worm of doubt persisted in my mind and I could not eliminate it.

My doctor scheduled another EEG test to verify the results of the first. She said that maybe the irritant dysrhythmic alterations were a consequence of my still-developing brain. So, another test would be the best thing to do. If that one was the same, other steps would be taken. A couple of days later, they did the second EEG, and the results were the same – irritant dysrhythmic alterations.

I thought maybe I had done something wrong. Maybe the waves in my head were altered because of the excitement that day. I had wanted to do the test right so much. But after hearing the exact same result, I was badly shaken! There was no logical explanation for this. My mind could not find any reasonable consolation. The doctor claimed that a further examination of my brain was needed, because this result indicated a brain disorder, particularly epilepsy or another seizure syndrome.

As if the given circumstances were not bad enough! My symptoms were already sufficiently hard and draining to deal with, I did not need epilepsy or other seizures in my life. Slowly, but surely, the situation caused an overload in my brain and body. First, battling my symptoms daily; then, not being able to study and worrying about my frequent absences from school; and on top of all that, my doctors could not find the problem. I was done! My general thoughts were *let's get this over and done with. I am fed up with all of this. I cannot deal with this situation. It is too hard, draining and above all stressful.*

My neurologist sent me for a CT scan[6] to get better, clearer results. Everything was happening in a chain reaction, so we did not have time to think about bad outcomes or negativity. The CT appointment was scheduled for 3 March 2003, at eight o'clock. I remember feeling happy to be missing out on a big German language test that day. If only someone could have warned me about the distressing events in the future, I would have opted for the test instead.

Although I had told Mum 'I think I have a brain tumour' after the first EEG, my initial thoughts were miles away from anything

---

[6] A computed tomography (CT) scan creates a two or three-dimensional image of any structure in the body.

being wrong with my brain. My whole system was overloaded and had had enough of everything. Yes, I was still shaken and astonished, but that overloaded state made me think calmly and reasonably. I felt flat. Everything was even to me, so I was not concerned at all. I was in for an ugly surprise. On second thoughts, maybe I should have been worried. But what purpose would that have served?

On the day of my CT scan, all three of us got up early—Mum and Dad to have their morning ritualistic coffee in peace, and me to watch them. The morning of my CT scan, I woke up happily, thinking the examination would be quick like the others and the rest of the day I would be free to thank my lucky stars. I had a very big, important exam that day. Everything in it was about German grammar, the part of German language I detested!

At 7:30 a.m. Mum and I headed for the hospital, while Dad went to his workshop. It was a fifteen to twenty-minute drive, but we wanted to arrive early. We sat down and waited for the procedure to start. The whole CT procedure lasted five minutes, then I was out in the waiting room. When the procedure finished so quickly, I was thrilled – finally something good! *I am on a roll, this morning!* Usually, the procedures and waiting for the results dragged on, a never-ending story. My mum and I were calm, expecting a normal result.

Suddenly, the waiting room door was wide open. A doctor and two nurses walked towards us. I will never forget what the doctor said, nor the way she said it. It was though someone had emptied a freezing cold bucket of water on me and rejoiced in doing so. 'We have a little issue. You should be admitted to the hospital', she said, with a smile on her face.

A brain tumour was a little issue? And when you say 'hospitalisation', would you say it with a smile? Outrageous! An animal would be treated with more respect, kindness, and compassion. All of this from a person who deals with these situations daily. If you do not have even an ounce of humanity in you, at least fake it. I was not a VIP. I did not expect special treatment, but I was – I am – a person with feelings and emotions. What is the big fuss over cancer anyway? Why do people overreact? It is just something you can die of! Maybe she thought those with medical degrees are immune from it. My astonishment at her behaviour overwhelms me.

The greatest cruelty is our casual blindness to the despair of others.

My mum and I just stood and stared at her. After some time, we came to our senses and said, 'What? Where?' We were blown away. Words were stuck.

As ordered by the doctor, we rushed to my neurologist – same hospital, different ward – with a million questions. *What is it? Is it something serious? Why hospitalisation?* When we arrived at the neurologist's office, she immediately started talking.

'Yes, unfortunately Tihana has a brain cyst[7]. Its official name is medulloblastoma fossae cranii posterior. It is half water and half hard formation. It is exceptionally large – six cm by four cm – and it is in the cerebellum[8]. Children ordinarily get it, but there is a one percent chance that adults get it too.'

At first, I was furious when I found out that 'the little issue' was a brain tumour. I needed a long time to overcome the anger, rage, and fury I felt for those words and for the one who uttered them. But now, as time has passed, I only feel sadness and grief.

---

[7] A cyst is a sac-like pocket of tissue that can grow anywhere in the body and is usually filled with fluid or air. Most cysts are benign.

[8] The cerebellum is the part of the brain that receives information from the sensory systems and spinal cord, and then regulates motor movements. The cerebellum coordinates voluntary movements such as posture, balance, coordination, and speech, resulting in smooth and balanced muscular movements.

Disbelief, too. How could someone act like that? Where is the humanity? Compassion? Apart from feeling furious, I was gob-smacked. Out of billons of people on this planet, I am in that one percent that get it later in life. Bad or maybe rotten luck. I was speechless!

The neurologist tried to sugar-coat the story as much as she could. She even avoided calling it a tumour by calling it a cyst instead, but nothing helped. I was crushed. I did not know what to say or do, so I just stared at her as she continued.

'The best thing you can do now is to come and stay in the hospital so that we can monitor you and operate as soon as possible. We advise you not to move too much because the tumour is pressing against a tubule in the brain which drains cerebro-spinal fluid[9]. If you move around too much that would cause hydrocephalus[10] and we would have to operate immediately. We would have to embed a small pump in your brain to stop the accumulation of CSF. This would be done before the operation to remove the tumour. That would delay things and we don't have time to waste.'

I kept staring at her and nodding, hoping all of it was a bad dream. From the moment of learning my diagnosis, I retreated into my safe place. All sorts of thoughts ran through my head. Bad thoughts. For a brief instant, a good thought crossed my mind: *maybe the doctor who gave me the results was using anxiety drugs, so she mixed up the results.* That would explain everything.

---

[9] Cerebrospinal fluid (CSF) is a clear, colourless fluid found in the brain and spine.
[10] Hydrocephalus is an abnormal accumulation of cerebrospinal fluid in the brain that can be fatal.

There I was, playing out the whole funny/tragic scenario in my head, when the words 'it's urgent' brought me back to reality. She gave me one last instruction before we left.

'We are preparing a room for you here at the neurology ward. Go home quickly, pack up only the essentials and remember do not jump or hop around because it's dangerous.'

Is it, really? I still did not realise what all the fuss was about. Things were clear from her explanation, but I was in denial.

'Before you go, I've arranged a meeting for you with our head neurosurgeon. He's free now, so you can visit him and arrange everything regarding the operation.'

If I had known what he was going to say, I would never have gone. My neurologist spoke so highly of him. She gave me the impression I was going to speak to the Pope himself. I am still having a hard time understanding why this 'Pope' was so mean? *Highly concealed hope slasher!*

The neurosurgeon was nice at first. He really did reassure me and made me think that not everything was so dark and that the sun would come out again. But as he kept blabbering on, my fears rose. He explained how it was an awfully bad situation and that meaningful recovery was unlikely. The tumour would be extremely hard to remove. Because of this a lot of healthy cells would be damaged. We can only hope that the tumour has not spread, because if has… In his experience, the outcome for this sort of tumour was either being a vegetable for the rest of my life or death. Rage consumed me, so I wanted to ask him whether I should prepare myself for the cemetery. Or maybe I should put myself out of my misery to begin with? Mum somehow detected this and stopped me.

After the meeting, we were sad, hopeless, and drained. We were helpless. Many scenarios played out in my head and none of them was positive, and I doubt any positive ones played in my mum's head. That man destroyed any hopes of survival or a positive outcome whatsoever. His approach was more than outrageous. I had not anticipated, nor hoped that he would say everything would be all fine and dandy. But this? When I received that diagnosis, my initial thoughts were not *this will be a piece of cake*, but his words were scary and demoralising. There was not even one word of beating the cancer, and God forbid that he said anything about possibly moving on after this. I do not even want to think what he does with patients who have a worse diagnosis than me. Give them the seventh sacrament? Is it possible that he directs those people to the nearest cemetery? It is a disgrace that sick people are treated this way.

The doctors filled my traumatic path with horrible situations, which were only supplemented by even worse ones. They could have reassured me by telling me there's a big fight ahead, but I will survive; even lying, telling me a big fat lie would have made me feel better. It could have given me hope. My already sad and traumatic path was embittered further because of the doctor's persona.

Thankfully, I have been hospital-free since coming to Australia for the second time, but my episodes with doctors make me look down on them to the point of nearly detesting them. I realise a book should not be judged by its cover, but the scars that are imprinted on my body are in my brain too. And the brain cannot disregard that some scars were caused by doctors.

A perfect name for this doctor is Doctor Wipe-Out. Truth be told, he deserves a much worse name. I think that name prepares the patients for what lies in front of them. Preparation is key! Without it, you are doomed. Seriously, he approaches you and you think *I am home safe* when you are standing at the threshold of hell.

A part of me cannot forget that horrible day I was diagnosed, and the other part will not forget it. I cannot because it left a permanent stain. This stain has two bad characteristics. First, it is not present for several days and then pops up out of the blue. Something reminds me – a picture of the brain, an illness, doctors. Second, I cannot forget because I have long-term psychological issues that stick to me like a leech. They are unwilling to leave me in peace.

To be truthful, I am not entirely comfortable letting go of them. A part of me would like to move on and continue with my life. But I am holding back. A voice in my head warns me that I cannot let go of what happened. If I stop thinking about the tumour, it may come back because it is not getting enough attention! To stay medically and mentally healthy, I cannot forget the tumour. It must be on my mind 24/7. I read somewhere that if a person truly asks for peace and oblivion, they can gain it. Maybe my request was not genuine enough. Maybe something happened between my heart and peace. Maybe it is easier said than done. Maybe the only people who can achieve peace and oblivion are people like Deepak Chopra, Wayne Dyer or Louise Hay. Or is it possible that all these maybes are just excuses? I truly hope the day comes when I go twenty-four hours without remembering my diagnosis. A day when I will be able to completely remove the traces of sorrow, pain, despondency and grief that diagnosis brought me.

On the other hand, I am guilty of playing the victim by not moving on, by staying in the same spot and not proceeding with my life. Stagnation is permissible during illness, but my situation is not like that anymore. Yet, I still find myself playing my favourite game. It is true that time heals everything. My physical wounds have mostly healed. My psychic wounds are healing slowly. But the past keeps haunting me. It is not so often now, but it is still there, hiding in the shadows. So much time has passed since that day, and I still feel like an ostrich with its head in the sand. Sometimes it is as if I am completely ignorant towards life, not caring for anything. Being blind, with vision and not wanting to use my gift! The main thing is that I have not overcome all that has happened and maybe that is why I refuse, on some level, to move on. Maybe I need to tell my story to receive closure and move on. Sharing the pain and sorrow buried deep inside might propel me out of this illness cycle.

It seems to me that when you conquer something, even bigger issues erupt. Do not get me wrong, I am incredibly grateful to be alive and well, but learning what can re-ignite the illness has left me in a perpetual state of worry. I cannot stop myself from constantly thinking this is so dangerous, I should not be doing this if I want to stay healthy, or I should not be eating that. It is a never-ending story, which has sadly developed into a way of life. Day in, day out, my thoughts revolve around what not to eat, acid and alkaline foods, my time spent watching TV, time spent on the computer, and mobile phone radiation. The truth is I have turned into a control freak. Not willingly or intentionally, but nonetheless, it makes my life extremely hard and exhausting. This also explains why I can't and won't let go. Fear keeps me from forgetting and moving on.

It has been eleven years since my diagnosis. There has not been a single day where a question like *Am I doing the right thing by watching TV? Is eating this food good for me? Will the radiation from my mobile phone and computer cause another one?* has not arisen. I am consumed by and stuck on these questions. It's clear to me that prevention is necessary and essential in my case, but my doing so is overwhelming. In justifying myself, I can only state **once bitten, twice shy**.

5

Family Ties

◇

What one does is what counts. Not what one had the intention of doing.

~**Pablo Picasso**

*M*eanwhile, my dad was going through a hell of his own. *We all have our own personal hell!* On the day of the CT scan, Mum and I went to the hospital, and Dad went to his workshop in a village near Osijek called Ivanovac.

That morning, around nine o'clock, my aunt got a call from one of her friends. That friend was an intern in the neurology ward in Osijek Hospital at the time. She knew something was wrong with me but did not know what. Immediately after that phone call, my aunt called my dad.

'What's going on with Tihana?'

My dad did not have a clue about what was going on. He was totally caught off guard. Naturally, it shook him up because the question was not asked in a calm manner; my aunt was in panic. Therefore, all my dad could assume were bad things – a big variety of them. His thoughts were set at levels: bad, worse and worst.

A subtle way to ask, wouldn't you think so? My dad, as a self-employed carpenter, had a crazy schedule, so she could have assumed he was not with us in the hospital. Didn't she consider that he might not know? Didn't it cross her mind that he needed a much gentler approach? Receiving such uncertain news brought nothing but worry and agitation to him. I know her intentions were good, but calling without knowing the problem and freaking him out? That is her brother! *Most people do not listen with the intent to understand; they listen with the intent to reply.*

After the doctor's diagnosis and the unpleasant meeting with Dr Wipe-Out, we headed to the car where I could calmly call Dad and tell him about my diagnosis. Of course, before calling him, Mum and I needed to collect ourselves and exit that crying stage! Not knowing anything about the bombshell he received earlier, I tried to break it to Dad gently. The news was bad, I agreed, but there was no time to cry, mourn or wonder how it happened. It was time for action, big-time action!

After that, we all met up at home where we had to tell my grandmother the news. That was an even harder task. At that time, I can safely say that she was an alcoholic. She occasionally had sane periods and times where she wanted to quit. Unfortunately, it was no longer a psychological need. It had become physical. Her body was accustomed to it. Even she, when no alcohol was present, realised alcohol was not good for her. But sadly, she could not cut it off. So, given her state, this news might cause her to fall off the wagon completely. *Here's to alcohol! The rose-coloured glasses of life.*

We carefully explained it to her, and she took it rather well, or so I thought. She seemed strong, supportive and determined, but it was on the outside. On the inside, it was a completely different story. Any shred of sanity or self-control had gone out the window. She became consumed by alcohol—a sad thing for her and for me. Had she hung in there, she would have been with us much longer. She was my sole living grandparent. It would have been wonderful if I had had her support and helping hand. It was so hard to watch her wane, but the biggest burden was on Mum. She was torn between her mother and me. It was so stressful and agonising for Mum, and the bad thing was that she held it all inside. I am so grateful my mum is still herself after all that happened.

I began packing for the hospital. Despite the situation, the atmosphere in the house was peaceful. After two hours, we went to the hospital. Since I like to drive around, Dad drove the scenic route to the neurology ward. We were talking all the way when a thought smacked me across the face: *I am going to die!* It was the first time I was horrified by what could happen. I started crying. Both of my parents questioned what was going on.

I asked them, 'What will happen if I die?'

Now, I understand that question troubled them even more, but I had to get my thoughts out in the open because they were driving me crazy. Neither one of them could have given me an answer, but I needed consolation. A word of comfort, to maybe shine some light in that hole I had fallen in.

My father urged me not to think that way and keep on fighting to overcome this. He said, 'Everything will be ok. You must think positively! The cards you have been dealt are awful. You probably even think they are not fair, but they are dealt and the only thing you can do is play them the best you can. Many people have battled with cancer and conquered it. You are not the first and you are not going to be the last. Nobody is saying the battle will be easy and fun. There will be tears. Pain. Frustration. And you and the two of us will feel a hell of a lot more emotions. Life is sometimes hard but remember that a positive state of mind makes it easier. You don't know the outcome of your life but that's the beauty of it, and life being beautiful makes it worth living despite all its faults.'

After hearing him say that, I felt hope. It was like I was renewed. It is well known worldwide that a merry heart does good like medicine. I knew it was going to be hard and that I would want to give up, but from then on, I really thought I could beat the tumour, and even grow from it. I was a fighter and would not stop until the end. My greatest fuel were my guardian angels – my parents, Mirela and Zvonimir, combined with the fact that quitting was not an option. I thought it would be ungrateful and malicious if I gave up, having the unconditional support and backup from my parents. I am not saying this to show myself as Miss Goody-Two-Shoes. My true stance is that is morally wrong, careless, and negligent to stop with something when you have any kind of backup. Mine was particularly good!

6

Osijek Hospital

◇

People are trapped in history, and history is trapped in them.

~**James Baldwin**

*W*hen we arrived at the hospital, the ward I was supposed to be in looked horrible. The whole hospital consisted of several different buildings, some high, some low and some almost insignificant. This one was a high building and had four levels. It was old and rustically built, not appealing at all. They had renewed the façade of the building recently, but that did not help. *Now it just looks like a huge white deathbed!* A hell house, but inside it was much worse. A nurse showed me down a long, dark corridor. My room was poorly lit with one big window looking towards the street, a big crucifix on the wall, one bed and a bedside table. It was a cold room without any consolation or hope. *Maybe they* *got their ideas for decoration from a prison, but then the room would have had a toilet.*

The entire hospital premises were depressing. It did have a park and one shop, without any ornaments. Nothing was nicely decorated. A truly depressing place! In my personal view, the hospital gave the vibe of death. Well, maybe not death but surely the place was not remedial, reparative, therapeutic or health-giving.

The nurse helped me settle into my room aka prison cell. The thought never entered my mind at the time, but now looking back, it almost seemed like a death preparation room. It was so depriving, denying a person any positive outcome, any hope that the future will be bright. Thank God, I did not realise this at the time. I think that would have destroyed my will to fight. Upon reflection, I argue why should it be that way? Why should a person let external situations and environments affect their willingness to fight? *Monsters do not sleep under your bed: they scream in your head.*

From that moment, all my feelings and emotions became numb, as if it was all an illusion and it was not happening to me. My initial thought was that this problem is bothering me now and it would soon pass. I knew surgery was necessary – not to stay alive, but because my doctor said so. Because of this numbness I thought this must-have operation would be routine and that nothing would change with my body. I refused to think or overthink because I did not want to let this place I was in, my diagnosis, or my other circumstances tear me down. Also, the numbness worked in my favour. *Like intoxication without narcotics!* So, I continued to keep myself busy – reading, studying, doing cross-word puzzles – all the things that made me happy, interested and content. We have a saying in Croatia, 'Iron rusts if not used. Still water grows stagnant. The power of the mind is weakened by inactivity'. Looking back, I was not worried at the time. I could not be. I just blocked everything. In my opinion that was the right thing to do. It was a defence mechanism. Consuming myself with thoughts of the illness, the operation and death would not help me fight against the tumour at all.

One thing that helped me at that time was my poor knowledge of the tumour. I did not know what the operation would bring or what side effects I would experience. The aftermath was totally unknown to me. I assumed after the operation everything would go back to normal. When the testing was ongoing, I saw many people who had had different brain tumour operations. They seemed reasonably okay. Yes, they had issues, but nothing compared to my outcome. I was better off not knowing. Otherwise, it would have been difficult. It is not easy to confront someone with the fact that you are able to walk into the hospital and may come out in a wheelchair. But change is inevitable, progress is optional. It entirely depends on us, what we do, how we approach and accept difficulties in life. There is no point in denying or blocking events. Accept them and learn how to turn them into something good. I know it is easier said than done but trust me it is possible. When you think about it, our only option is to accept whatever comes to us. Either carry on or die! Like my dad always says: **get busy living or get busy dying**.

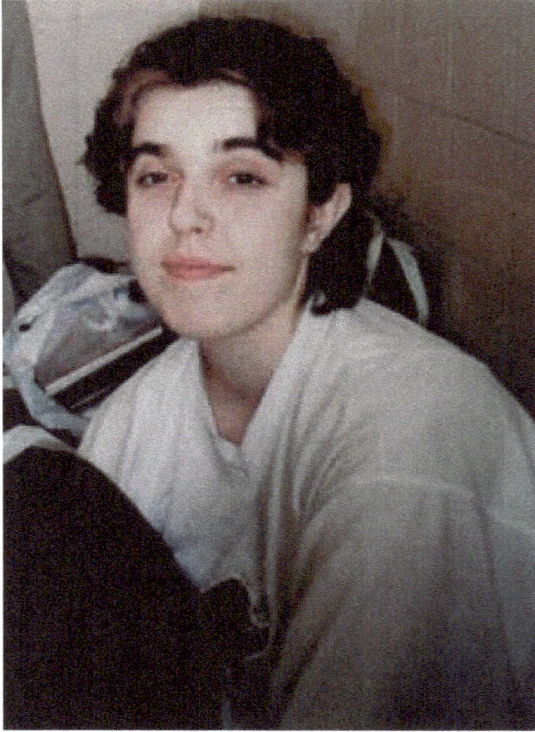

Waiting at Osijek Hospital

My parents visited me frequently. Thank God for that! From time to time, they would stumble upon the head of the neurology ward. She advised them to take me abroad because the operation would be better and faster. A head doctor of a ward insecure about the performance of the hospital she works in. What does that spell? Mayday! Mayday!

7

Dr Dreadful

◇

The death of hope and love is far worse
than death itself.

–C. J. Anderson

While I was waiting for my operation, my family and I were miserable. We cried for most of the day, them at home and me in the hospital. The diagnosis crushed all of us – my mum, my dad, my grandmother and me. To be honest I am not entirely sure what was going on with me then. Yes, I had been shot down from my path and was in panic, terrified, but a part of me was in that limbo state where you are just numb. Contradictory, I know, but bad thoughts rained on me. I panicked about dying, being left in bed for the rest of my life like a vegetable or something similar. It was dark in my mind and I thought that no light would shine on me ever again. Generally, disregarding those black moments, my stance was *let it be over with so everything could return to normal.*

Prior to this health scare, my knowledge of brain tumours, or cancer for that matter, was non-existent. My overall attitude was that this will be conquered and that is it. There'd be no side effects. Nothing would follow on once they have extracted that tumour. Relying on that, I wanted to have the operation immediately. It is almost like imagining someone literally getting in my head and shooting the unwanted guest there. *Too many American movies!*

The next day, my mum and my dad decided to do something, with no time to waste. The goal was to find a good neurosurgeon to operate. The phone was extremely active from 3 March until 8 or 9 March, as either my parents called someone, or someone was calling them. They were determined to find a neurosurgeon because, up until now, none of the doctors we'd seen could reassure them that everything would be alright, so that they could be at ease and relax. Their wanting to find someone who could do the job completely and successfully was a priority and essential. At the end of the day, this operation was not considered a routine procedure; it was an extremely risky endeavour. There were several reasons for this, but mainly because I would be seated rather than lying down throughout the operation. That is a very troublesome position in which a lot could go wrong but it is useful. The benefits of the seated position in neurosurgery include access to the neck and spine, and otherwise hard-to-reach parts of the brain. It also allows for improved venous and cerebrospinal fluid drainage, potentially lowering intracranial pressure. Out of many things that could go wrong, the major risk factor from the seated position is developing a gas embolism, where a bubble of gas enters the circulatory system, potentially causing a stroke or heart attack. Therefore, an expert was needed. In my opinion, my parents kept busy during this time because it helped them cope with the situation better.

After learning about the options in Osijek, Mum and Dad were not convinced that surgery on the local ward would yield a good outcome. One option was a neurosurgeon, Dr Angel, in Zagreb, Croatia's capital city. Unfortunately, almost all the doctors in Osijek claimed he was not working any more due to alcoholism and shaky hands. Basically, they said he had lost his touch. *Unbeknownst to the doctors in Osijek, his 'shaky' hands made it possible for me to tell you this story.*

While searching, my mother spoke to her cousin's wife who is a gynaecologist. She remembered a friend and colleague from university, a trained neurosurgeon – Dr Dreadful – working in Osijek's hospital. The gynaecologist contacted her friend Dr Dreadful to discuss my case, and if possible, schedule a meeting with him. *Enormous mistake!* A day later, she called us and told us when the meeting would take place. The gynaecologist was insistent that another doctor should be present, but she was working a hospital shift that day. Was it because Dr Dreadful would not believe our story?

My mother then remembered her other cousin who is an orthopaedist. He agreed to come to the meeting. I remained in hospital while my parents and Mum's cousin, the orthopaedist, attended the meeting.

The meeting went well at first. From the introductions, Dr Dreadful seemed okay, a pleasant man. But as they were talking about the operation and the risks involved, he became agitated. For no apparent reason, he adopted an 'I am the doctor, I know everything' persona.

My father asked, 'How many operations like this one have you performed?'

'What does it matter?' he replied.

My father started fuming. 'Well, it's brain surgery, not a finger operation, so it does indeed matter!'

After hearing that, the doctor grew even more agitated. My father was thinking if he is agitated and nervous just because of an innocent question, how the hell will he react if a problem in the operating room occurs? To me and my family a brain operation seemed extremely dangerous. As far as I was concerned, the brain was the king of the body. One should be cautious of it and treat it with respect. Everything starts and ends with it. If the brain does not work, then you are as good as dead.

Dr Dreadful continued explaining the procedure, how it was conducted in a seated position, which alone was difficult on the body: 'Few people could withstand that. It's exceedingly difficult, very high risk. It offers an incredibly low chance of survival, and even if someone lives, the aftermath could kill him.'

Maybe I should have committed suicide to spare him the misery of conducting such an impossible procedure. To this day I cannot understand why someone would give him the possibility, let alone the qualification, to be a neurosurgeon.

My father's second question was, 'How is the hospital equipped?'

Dr Dreadful responded, 'Like any other hospital in the United States.'

Automatically, my dad replied, 'Then why did our former president go abroad when he was ill and needed an operation?'[11]

That question was the drop that tipped the glass. Dr Dreadful exploded. He was emitting gas and it was toxic! 'You are being

---

[11] Franjo Tudman was the first president of Croatia and served from 1990 until his death in 1999. Controversially, he went to Texas for cancer treatment in 1995.

very, very rude and disrespectful, Mr Babic Your daughter is battling for her life. She is in an extremely dangerous situation with slim odds. We should operate as soon as possible and not worry about our former president. He is dead and buried! This is a profoundly serious operation. We cannot guarantee a positive outcome. It is a dangerous operation in a half-lying, half-sitting position. You should concern yourself with the outcome, and – if the operation is successful – the aftermath.'

His speech was full of repetition and questionable success. By this stage, my parents were terrified. It was as if I was sentenced to death and the only thing in question was when I would die.

Then my father asked, 'Are you trying to tell us that our daughter has one foot in the grave?'

The doctor's face changed from dark pink to dark red. He was so enraged that he rushed out of the room screaming, 'Goodbye!', and slammed the door on his way out.

My father commented that he would not let that doctor operate if he was the last neurosurgeon on earth. Doctors carry an extremely large amount of responsibility. If an accountant or an architect make a mistake, in most cases, it can be resolved. They can afford a mistake here and there in their careers, but doctors do not have that privilege. When they mess up, the price is high. A doctor's mistake can forever mark a person's life or be fatal.

One good thing about the meeting was that I was not present, because I believe that man would have totally extinguished any hope of me conquering this successfully. I am not even including the devastation, misery and hopelessness he would leave in my life. Thank heavens I was not present. Even Dr Wipe-Out, the doctor whom I initially saw, was pleasant compared to Dr Dreadful. When a person comes across doctors like that, it makes you wonder why that person practises medicine in the first place. What is their purpose in doing so? My path was filled with so many awful doctors that they cannot all be listed. It was true agony going through everything without reassurance, trust or security. In every medical situation, one needs someone who not only knows what they are doing, but who is positive and does not scare you to death with your diagnosis.

This incident, along with the Dr Wipe-Out disaster and other situations leading up to now, made my battle even more painful. These moments were just the beginnings of doctors' vanity, egoism, arrogance, boastfulness, and coldness. Sadly, through everything that happened throughout my cancer journey I have learnt that the doctor is important; the patient and their illness are irrelevant.

8

Peer Support

◇

Friendship isn't a big thing, it's a million little things.

~Paulo Coelho

A lot of relatives and friends came to see me in the hospital. Some did it out of remorse, pity or fear that the same thing might happen to them. I believe that this last listed reason is truer than the first two. Sadly, my only true family and friends are my parents. They were always one hundred percent behind me, forming a safety net. They were constantly by my side. Others were there when it was convenient for them, but when it was not, they mysteriously vanished. It's sad, depressing, and brings tears to my eyes to remember.

But one visit was so unexpected and nearly impossible that it surprised me – my class. From thirty-one students in my class, twenty-six came, including my professor. She must have sacrificed her school hours to come with the students. The gesture revealed unspoken words of caring and selflessness that truly meant a lot to me. We could not go outside onto the hospital grounds because I risked hydrocephalus (a build-up of CSF fluid in the brain) if I moved. Also, I was on a drip, but it was lovely all the same. Initially, I was astonished. Who was I to receive a wonderful gift like this? They all had to cut school by an hour or more to get here. Have I become a VIP? For a moment I forgot all about the illness, the negativity and the sorrow, and acted like a completely normal teenager. We talked, laughed, joked, and my surroundings became irrelevant. It felt like we were in an actual classroom. I cannot explain the emotions that ran through me. All of them were so good, some even went into overload. My heart was full, and during those forty-five minutes everything bad vanished into thin air. In that time, I was cancer-free, a healthy teenager, and it felt extraordinarily good.

When my professor said that it was time for them to leave, all the negativity returned.

In an instant, everything went dark. There was no hope. I had tears in my eyes. It hurt! It was like that song 'It's All Coming Back to Me Now' by Celine Dion. But I did not finish crying the instant they left when everything became silent. Instead of keeping all the memories close to my heart, they haunted me. The uncertainty of the situation compared to the memories of school, teenage, normal life made me depressed and incredibly sad. My circle of friends was not broad, but it greatly diminished when everyone heard about my illness. This visit really woke me up. It moved me from my trauma to a wonderful place where everything was happy, joyous and exciting. I think that was the reason my mood dropped so hard that it hurt. I was not sure whether I would experience those emotions ever again. It felt like I was sentenced to death and I was just waiting for my verdict to be carried out. *Awful!* This was one more episode of bad thoughts that rained on me. I knew they were going to stop, and I would return to that limbo state. In the limbo state, I was okay. Everything was calm, unemotional and collected. My interest in maths, crosswords and reading was enough and it kept me busy. My mind was occupied and that was important.

Visiting hours in the hospital were in the morning and afternoon. That day, my class and professor came earlier, and my friend Marija came to see me later. Her grandparents lived across the street from my house, so over time we had become close. We shared a lot, something I did not have with many people. As we grew older, I guess our friendship reached the point where I felt able to open up to her and tell her my true thoughts and feelings. So, as I was in that limbo state, I told her, 'I do not care what happens if I live or die. I just want everything to be over and done with!'

Saying that to someone else helped me relieve my soul. It gave me a feeling of letting go of a choking burden. It was pure liberation. This may indeed seem like an overstatement or foolery, but those words coming out of my mouth freed me. I was transformed by those sentences. From that point, I was not in excruciating fear. My whole perception of this distressful event has changed. Those words became my goal though everything: *I do not care for the outcome, just let it pass!*

On my health journey, some of my relatives and closest friends kept away from me like I had the plague. That devastated me. I do not hold anything against them, but when I see those people now, it brings back painful memories. It is a permanent stain. I have tried to eliminate these feelings, but they do not go away. Maybe I do not want them to go. But I think their mask of great friendship has been removed, which is a good thing. It is a painful realisation that not many so-called friends hang around. The saying that misfortune tests friends and reveals enemies is absolutely true. They did not become my enemies, but they tarnished my life in terms of me holding anger, bitterness and resentment towards them. I have managed to let go of those bad emotions now, but a bitter taste in my mouth arises every time I see them. There is an old saying in Croatia, which explains it perfectly: A wolf changes its fur, but its nature stays the same. The thing I can't understand is why do people want to continue our so-called friendship? Do they have amnesia? Maybe they thought I was a toddler so I would forget. *Strange!*

9

Dr Angel

◇

We must accept finite disappointment, but never lose infinite hope.

~Martin Luther King Jr.

I was in hospital and waiting for surgery. By now it was crystal clear that Osijek was out of the picture for the operation. The search for a surgeon needed to be widened to Zagreb or even abroad. It was a difficult situation because on the one hand, it was urgent and on the other, there was no one to operate. Well, no one we considered fit for the job, anyway. We had only met with two neurosurgeons, I am aware of that, but witnessing their feelings and emotions combined with our own terrifying thoughts did not reassure us that others would be much different.

With this in mind, Dad searched the internet in the hope of finding a good neurosurgeon. As he searched, he stumbled upon a clinic for brain tumours in Cologne, Germany. But later he discovered that they do not operate. Nevertheless, he did find an internationally renowned Slovenian neurosurgeon who was an exceptionally good and highly praised doctor. Dad decided to give him a call to see if he was able to do the operation. It was a semi-struggle to get the doctor on the phone, but eventually he picked up. When he heard my diagnosis, he was willing to operate, but was puzzled. Why him?

He said, 'You would have to spend a lot of money to have the treatment in Slovenia, when everything could be done in Croatia. Your country has a remarkably successful neurosurgeon. The best in south-eastern Europe.

My dad was puzzled and confused. The doctors in Osijek had told us our only option was to go to some other country. Dad asked, 'Who?'

The answer was Dr Angel. This confused my father even more. From what he had heard, Dr Angel had stopped working years ago. The doctors in Osijek hospital had told us he was an alcoholic with shaky hands. As it turned out, Dr Angel was indeed still operating and very successfully for that matter. Perhaps the doctors we spoke to in Osijek were envious and jealous. I am not surprised by this at all, judging from the doctors we dealt with. My health crisis really showed me how vain doctors are. In my opinion, Dr Wipe-Out and Dr Dreadful were egotistical, boastful, arrogant, basically vainglorious. Aren't they supposed to help people and give them hope, not satisfy their childish egos?

We needed to get in touch with Dr Angel. That turned out to be mission impossible without a connection. *Perhaps if Tom Cruise had been available everything would have been easier.* After some research online, Dad found out that Dr Angel worked in a hospital called Rebro, in Croatia's capital Zagreb. At the time, he was the head of neurosurgery in Rebro, and head of another hospital in Zagreb, called Šalata. When my father called the doctor, his personal secretary said that he was incredibly busy, and that the best thing to do would be to come to the hospital and wait. Unfortunately, that was the only way.

In the meantime, Mum and Dad saw a good friend of ours. Our families were friends because I'd gone to primary school with her son. As her son and I became good friends, our families grew closer as well. She told my Dad she had heard what happened to me, and she was wondering what she could do to help. Her name was well known in Osijek and Zagreb because she was the secretary of a well-known political party in Croatia, the Democratic Centre. That meant she had a lot of connections to influential people.

My dad said, 'If you could somehow get in touch with Dr Angel, it would be wonderful. I'm not into politics, but if you succeed, I'll become a member of Democratic Centre.'

She answered, 'Leave it to me, I'll see what I can do!'

In the meantime, my parents decided to travel the 280 kilometres from Osijek to Zagreb and test their luck at Rebro. They had to be at the hospital early in the morning if they wanted a positive outcome. Now another issue appeared – my medical records. Of all my records, my parents only had the CT scans. They needed more than that. My parents came to visit me at Osijek Hospital that afternoon and decided to gather my medical reports at the same time. This turned out to be one of the many stumbling blocks in my battle. As they visited me, they went to the head doctor's office. At first, she was wonderful. They were talking about my situation, and my dad said that he had found a doctor in Zagreb, so he needed my medical reports.

Upon hearing that she freaked! 'Mr Babic, I'm amazed. I thought you were a reasonable man! By now both of you should know that Tihana is in an extremely dangerous situation. Too much movement is not advised. It is prohibited! Your intention is dangerous and injudicious. All the care she needs is provided here, so she doesn't need to go elsewhere!'

Irritated, Dad replied, 'She's our daughter and we're doing what should have been done days ago. I doubt very much that you will be upset if she dies! So please give us the medical reports, and we'll be out of here as soon as possible.'

After that she eased up and gave my dad all the medical documentation. Mum and Dad returned to my room visibly tired but content. We did not discuss anything because anyone could walk in. It is not like we had not got used to difficulties and setbacks with doctors. But seriously, it seemed like she was stalling. If my situation was so urgent, why was she delaying the process? Does one try to prove how good a doctor they are, or how efficient their hospital is by delaying surgery? And, if a doctor flippantly changes their mind about things, does that make them reliable in emergency situations? I think not.

Mum and Dad told me their plan and asked me to hang in there. As soon as they got home, Mum and Dad quickly packed up. The next day, they arrived at the neurosurgery ward at Rebro Hospital in Zagreb. It was overflowing with people, even though it was early in the morning. They waited. It began to seem like a lost cause. Then, seven hours later, Dr Angel's nurse announced that everyone who was waiting for him should go home. He would not be seeing anybody else that day, other than the vice ambassador of Macedonia and the Babic family. Everybody else, disappointed and angry, left. Then she said, 'Mr Babic, Dr Angel will be waiting for you at the Šalata hospital within an hour. Bring all the medical documentation you have, and he will see you.'

My friend's mum had succeeded! God bless her! Later, we found out how. Being a secretary in the Democratic Centre, she contacted one of the leading men in the party. This man was a close friend of Dr Angel. She told him about my case, and he agreed to contact him. I do not know how or why. I was a stranger to this person. I guess when someone is genuinely good, they are good to anyone, known or unknown. Anyway, thanks to her, we managed to get in contact with Dr Angel. I am forever thankful to her and her family. There is a Croatian saying: No matter how distant you are, some people are linked to you for the rest of your life.

While my parents were in Zagreb, I was resting at the hospital back in Osijek. I was not terrified, worried, or freaking out. On the contrary, my hours passed peacefully. The main thing I focused on was that all of this would pass, that one day, I would return to my everyday, regular life. I enjoyed technical drawing and solving mathematical problems, so I filled my days doing that, basically preparing myself for university. I was in my final year of high school, and my electives were natural science and mathematics. I wanted to attend the Architectural University or University of Mechanical Engineering and Shipbuilding.

In the meantime, my parents headed to the Šalata hospital, but they had no idea how to get there. Problem one was that they needed to be there in an hour. Problem two was that they had rarely been to Zagreb, so the streets were a total enigma to them. My parents had driven to Zagreb in their own car, and everything they needed for the trip was packed in it – food, clothing, paperwork. Given that the car was needed, they could not use public transport or a taxi. Eventually, Dad decided to call a taxi that would lead them to the Šalata hospital and they would follow.

Šalata was a huge, blue hospital with big, curved windows. Pictures of it, prior to my surgery, amazed me. I did not know what it looked like inside, but outside it was beautiful. Later, my parents told me it was nice looking inside too. The neurosurgery ward was broad with a long corridor that led to the waiting room. My parents sat down and waited for the nurse to call them. They had been waiting for twenty minutes when all the doors in the long corridor opened. Everybody in the waiting room realised Dr Angel had arrived. Shortly after that, my parents were called in. He seemed like a major VIP because everyone got shook up when he entered the ward. Due to his diligence, we learnt immediately that he was strict and thorough in everything, not only his job. The staff were absolutely terrified of him.

The minute my parents saw him, both began crying. The man before them was peaceful, calm, reassuring. Just by seeing him, they knew the surgery would be a success. In the words of my parents, Dr Angel's persona gave the impression that he was one hundred percent confident in his abilities, skills, and performance. In their eyes, he was the right surgeon for me. That is why they cried.

After a couple minutes, Dr Angel said, 'Come on, stop crying! No time for that, we need to act.' When my parents composed themselves, they gave him the CT scan pictures and other medical reports. 'Yes, that unfortunately is a brain tumour. It needs to be urgently extracted or it could be fatal. It is big, so it must be removed quickly. The tumour is malignant, so it is cancerous. The cells can grow and spread to other parts of the body – namely areas around the brain and spinal cord.' Then, Dr Angel immediately grabbed a phone and reserved a bed for me for Monday morning. 'Don't worry about anything. She will be fine once the tumour is out. I know it is not easy, but you must be strong for her. Please bring her to Rebro on Monday before eight o'clock. Be vigilant, and don't let her move too much.'

After the meeting with Dr Angel, my parents headed home to Osijek so that they could arrange an ambulance to take me to Rebro Hospital for Monday morning. A huge burden had been lifted off their shoulders. They still did not know what the outcome would be, but their strength was renewed. They were hopeful for the first time in weeks. There was light at the end of the tunnel, and there was optimism and reassurance that everything would turn out alright.

I am not trying to convey that Dr Angel had magically made them believe that my cancer was child's play and could be removed easily, effortlessly. But his behaviour and approach had calmed them into thinking that this could be resolved and that I had a chance at life after all. There was no negativity or bad aspirations, assumptions, or affirmations. What delighted them most was the fact that he did not get agitated; he approached the tumour fearlessly and with confidence that he could completely remove it.

10

Ambulance Issue

◇

Happiness lies in the joy of achievement and the thrill of creative effort.

~Franklin D. Roosevelt

As my parents were driving back from Zagreb to Osijek, somewhere in the middle, Mum decided to organise the transport. She had to because the hospital in Osijek did not want anything to do with it. The moment my parents decided to transfer me to another hospital, the doctors at Osijek's neurological ward started playing dumb. They wanted me to stay so their doctors could do the surgery. They still did their ordinary rounds but that was pure courtesy. The neurosurgeons in the hospital would not operate, so they would not help me. *I'm lost for words!*

My mother remembered her cousin, the orthopaedist. She explained the situation to him, and he managed to organise a brand-new ambulance to take me to Rebro. Because of the risk of hydrocephalus, it was best to move me in an ambulance.

It was Friday night, and my inner state was not good. I was falling deeper and deeper into depression. Earlier, Mum and Dad came and told me the happy news, but after they left, I was all alone with my thoughts. Generally, the news made me smile and I was happy, but it did not keep me happy for long. My focus was on what was to happen now that the operation was set. I knew the only way to battle my illness was through this operation, but I was terrified of the whole process – the preparation for the operation, the operation itself and recovery. In the first stage, my worries were *what is going to happen? Will it hurt? How will they resolve hydrocephalus if it does occur?* When I think of these questions now, they seem as things that were completely out of my control, but at that time…

In the second stage, all my pounding thoughts were about the operation. Fearful assumptions that things would not go as planned. I also had negative thoughts that the operation would be cancelled for some reason.

And the third stage of my preoccupations focused on my state after the surgery. I did not have a clue that the aftermath would be so bad or that anything would change in my body. My expectations were minor things, not obvious at all. What worried me was that I would end up in bed for the rest of my life, in a vegetative state. This negative state was torturous to the point that I did not know where the end was. Was there an end to all of this?

And then my consolation arrived! My parents called. We talked, and my worries and fears disappeared. They gave me blissful medication in word form, and I returned to my normal state of being.

Saturday and Sunday passed, so I was off to Zagreb. The journey started at three a.m. on Monday morning. My mum and dad came to put all my things in our car. Mum and I were going in the ambulance, while Dad followed in our car. With relief, we arrived at Rebro in Zagreb. Nothing went wrong. No hydrocephalus, no nothing. Everything was in order. Now I just needed to stay calm and collected.

The hospital was different from the hospital in Osijek, but then I did not have time to wander around and see for myself. We entered the hospital and sat down in the waiting room for the nurse to call me. The moment she did, I was put in a wheelchair and she led me to my room. I settled down in my room and my parents stayed by my side all day. *A nice occurrence in a not-so-nice circumstance!* I was in Rebro Hospital, and everything was okay. The only thing left to do was wait for the main event.

11

Preliminary Arrangements

The difference between winning and losing is most often not quitting.

~Walt Disney

After putting all my stuff away in my new room in Rebro Hospital, I began to calm down. There were two other ladies with me in the room. Once I started chatting to them, the stress about the transfer and settling in vanished. They were genuinely nice. One was younger than me and the other was older. They cheered me up when I was down and vice versa. It was wonderful to have someone other than my parents to talk to. These girls were in similar situations to me, so they understood. Both had had a spinal operation, ending their torment. Only recuperation for them. *My torment still awaited!* They did not have any benign or malignant growths on their spines, only normal spinal issues that had to be operated on. That was the hard thing to bear:

they just needed to slowly move and exercise to get everything working again.

It was around six p.m., and my first visit from the doctors was just about to start. New doctors, new nurses, will it be different from the hospital in Osijek? Some doctor came. He got better acquainted with my situation. He found out some things from Dr Angel, but he needed more information in order to give me the right pre-operative instructions. That evening, I found out when the operation would take place and the procedure before the actual surgery. My operation was to take place the next day on Tuesday, 11 March 2003. There would be no eating or drinking for the rest of the evening, or tomorrow morning. My hair would be washed with a special disinfectant shampoo. They would have to shave off my hair where the incision was planned. The staff would administer an enema, so they could clear my bowels before the operation. Lastly, the doctor said, 'Your situation isn't pleasant but hang in there. Please try not to stress because you will not accomplish anything. Be calm and patient, and this will pass.' Such a wonderful change, a completely different approach from my previous doctors. Had they studied the same medicine?

The feeling that everything would end soon was great and I was happy about that. On the other hand, I was panicking and terrified about the whole procedure. I could not calm down because my brain would not let go of the anxiety. It played out different scenarios. Only a few had a positive outcome. *Could my body withstand the seated position? What if they did not have enough blood? What if I died on the table?* The 'what if' questions were infinite. The negativity hit me again, only two full days since my last outburst. This time, the feelings were more intense, more profound, and I thought I would go crazy. I could not get consolation from my parents; they were not with me. They were searching for accommodation, and I did not want to burden my roomies with my issues. So, it was up to me to rescue myself from that hole I had fallen into. I started contemplating what could help me.

In that moment it hit me: it is either this or alternative medicine. Pick or choose. Carefully, my mind started considering those two options. I concluded that alternative medicine is not what I would choose. The issue with that kind of medicine was that it did not make sense to me. I could not get myself to completely surrender to it. I do not think it is as powerful as conventional medicine. Then and there, I decided to give it my all and fight with my mind, body and soul. The plan was not to let this thing destroy me! I coached myself through it. The only option was to overcome my fear and stand up straight with my fighting gloves on! Immediately, the words of 'I'm a Survivor' by Destiny's Child played in my head.

My mind was made up. The fear did not go away entirely but I knew that this operation was a must-do to get on with my life, to surpass this. I could not surrender. I realised that all the fear, doubts and pain are temporary. All of that will pass. The one thing that would not pass is quitting. A person cannot quit and stay in the battle. When you quit it lasts forever! I did not want to 'live' day by day and witness my health deteriorating; I wanted to overcome the current state of my health.

12

Female Obstacles

◇

Pain is inevitable. Suffering is optional.

~Haruki Murakami

A few hours later, at around eight p.m., the emotional whirlpool slowly started to subside. Everything returned to normal. I kept on reassuring myself, to move my focus from negativity and redirect it towards my earlier decision: the operation was a must-do. No negotiation about that. The surgery was tomorrow, and I just needed to hang in there.

Around ten p.m., I was putting my things in the cabinet and preparing to go to bed, when, out of nowhere, I fainted. When I came to, everyone in the room, plus five or six nurses, was gathered around me. Everything was fine. The nurses measured my blood pressure, and it was extremely low, so that may have caused the fainting. It could also have been connected to the tumour, so the doctor who came to check on me ordered a nurse to accompany me wherever I went. Honestly, there were not a lot of places you could go in the hospital, so that was unnecessary in my opinion. But to some degree I could understand them. Had I got hurt while under their care, they would have been fined.

The next morning, after visiting the toilet, I was feeling kind of funny and I knew why – my period. *Bad, rotten luck!* This meant that everything said and planned was not going to happen. I did not know what my period would affect, but I was aware it had some consequences on the operation. When the doctors made their rounds, I found out what the repercussions were. The doctor told me that the operation would be postponed, due to the period issue. Operating while losing blood was dangerous; it would be additional loss. So, everything had to be postponed in order to prevent additional problems from happening. The procedure before the operation would take place on Thursday and the operation itself was moved to Friday.

My fear and all the negative energy behind the surgery subsided because of the postponement. But then, I was even more terrified of what the consequences would be. When my parents learnt the operation had been postponed, they panicked too. My mind buzzed with all sorts of questions. *How will I mentally survive the next three days? What can I do? How do I prevent negative thoughts? Will the operation have a positive outcome?* There was no way forward because of my period. That thought made everyone helpless. To mentally survive those next three days, I had to come up with something that could make time fly. Not just fly, but rocket fly. *If only 'Back to the Future' were not science fiction.*

On Wednesday morning, immediately after opening my eyes, I thought one day has passed positively; let's hope the next two follow. I decided to focus on the people around me to save me. No negativity, no doubts, no second thoughts. Truth be told, there was a big contradiction in my head. I knew the operation was a must-do, but I was still terrified of it and the outcome, which was making me reluctant to have it. I feared being in bed for the rest of my life or dying. I remembered the deal I made with myself, and how I would endure everything that comes. Yet, I could not seem to let time take its course. The dilemma persists!

My two roomies were with me, so I was not left by myself, crying about my circumstances. They were complete strangers and yet their words and actions showed otherwise. It seemed as if we had known each other for ages and really understood one another. Truly, beautiful people! Could not ask for more loving, reasonable, and joyous people. We talked a lot and shared our different life situations. Even though they were so good to me, I must admit I envied their situations. If I had any bad thoughts about either of them, may they all come back to me. I was jealous of their circumstances. I wanted to switch places with them just because their agony was over. Their surgeries had been successful, and they were recuperating. As I mentioned earlier, both had undergone spine operations. Their only visible problems were slow movement due to the surgical scarring, but other than that they were safely recovering. My agony was not knowing my outcome. I was physically functioning in that pre-operative state, but would I be the same afterwards? Or would I become a vegetable, even die? These were my fears, and I cannot condemn my roommates because they had dealt with theirs already, but still I was jealous. I envied them for quickly solving their issues, while the outcome of my issue remained unknown. I did not and do not apologise for my feelings. I am only human!

My parents visited me constantly. Thank God for that – though I am surprised the staff let them, given the strict hospital rules. The thought of so many people cheering me on made me stronger and helped me a lot. I can understand my mum and dad's support but everyone else, from the hospital personnel, nurses, doctors, my roomies? I was astonished! Quite the opposite of the hospital in Osijek. *Genuinely nice change!*

'Kindness in words creates confidence. Kindness in thinking creates profoundness. Kindness in giving creates love.'[12]

---

[12] Lao Tzu, Chinese philosopher

13

The Eve before the Operation

◇

The way I see it, if you want the rainbow, you got to put up with the rain.

~Dolly Parton

On Thursday morning's rounds, the doctors confirmed that the operation would take place at eight o'clock the following morning, and that all the preparations would be done that night. Only two days had passed since my mind, body and soul had come to a peaceful consensus about the surgery. Now, it seemed like everything had been thrown out the window. There was no time for a panic attack, but my mind was divided and could not stick to any decision. Both positive and negative thoughts tormented me. Even my crossword puzzles, books and magazines did not help. A few hours were left until the actual surgery and I could not stop stressing. I cannot say that I was consumed by negative thoughts or worries about bad outcomes, it was just that I was unable to calm down. What caused it was an enigma. My mind was going through a mix of emotions that could not be stopped.

The last round before the surgery took place at six p.m. The doctor told me the pre-operative procedures would start. From then on, I was not to eat or drink anything. Dinner would be served once the doctors' rounds finished. I could eat that and drink a bit of water, but afterwards any kind of food and drink was banned. The nurses would come in shortly to wash my hair with a special shampoo, and later an enema would be done to clear out my bowels. I would not get any medication tonight. Tomorrow morning, before they took me to theatre, I would get a tablet accompanied by an injection for the anaesthesia. Once all that was over, I would be set for the surgery.

The nurses came in minutes after dinner. They gave me the disinfectant shampoo, and I took a shower and washed my hair. I had done all the things required: only the enema awaited. Around eight p.m., a nurse came in to do it. It felt so uncomfortable. The water goes into your bowel and you must hold it in there if you can. When you cannot hold it anymore, you can poo. *Oh dear, it's awfully hard!* On top of that, the nurse stays by your side the entire time even when you poo. She could have at least stood in front of the bathroom door. I do not know why they left out shaving my head. Maybe they decided to do that right before they cut. Around nine p.m. and everything was done. Thank God! *Or so I thought.*

That night, maybe one hour later, an anaesthesiologist walked in the room and told me they needed to do one more thing. He said that they usually did this to patients under anaesthesia, but because I was such a good sport with the enema, he decided to hurry things up. Wasn't that a big ego boost? I could have dislocated my neck with my head held so high. I was so proud that I, Tihana Babic, was a good sport! That ego boost came crashing down like a house of cards once I realised what he was about to do.

He planned to insert a small tube into my arm with the help of a needle, and then push the tube through my neck, all the way down to my lungs. Was he freaking kidding? How? In my mind I was marching down the street with a protest placard in my hands, screaming, 'I WANT DRUGS! I WANT DRUGS! I WANT DRUGS!' But before I could utter the words, in one swift motion, the needle was in my arm. One detail he forgot to mention was that he would keep pushing the tube until it pointed down towards my stomach and he would be checking that with an X-ray. This was necessary so that the anaesthesia spread equally. As if I was not going through enough suffering and pain. Maybe he thought I was strong because I was so big? But I am not that strong. I am just fat, and that makes me look big! I desperately wanted to tell him that. We went back and forth from the X-ray room to make sure the placement was correct, and the third time was the charm. By midnight, all the procedures were finally concluded. I was drained from the last one. The enema and the anaesthesia procedure were the worst. The enema did not hurt: it was extremely uncomfortable. The anaesthesia procedure was both very painful and exceptionally uncomfortable – especially through the night. Hence why it is usually done under anaesthesia.

14

D-Day

〉

You can close your eyes to things you don't want to see, but you can't close your heart to things you don't want to feel.

~Johnny Depp

The surgery was on 14 March 2003. The day arrived and my feelings were all mixed up – hope, happiness, despair, grief. The feelings were changing just like on an audio player. The only issue was that I did not have the commands. So, the wanted emotions did not last long before the unwanted ones took over. That morning, while brushing my teeth, an overload of feelings hit me. I did not care about the outcome anymore. Yes, there was an ounce of fear left but generally my thoughts and feelings regarding all that was about to transpire were gone. All the worrying for tomorrow had taken its toll on me. The rush of different emotions from the time I was diagnosed up to now were taunting, depriving, exhausting. My body, mind and soul – my entire being – was in overdrive. Was this normal? Was this a safety firewall sent from above? I do not know what it was, but it felt like all the anguish, worry, overthinking, assumptions were enough. My body did not have the energy or the strength to deal with it anymore. I was done! It is a pity that all these feelings did not arrive earlier. They could have saved me a great amount of energy.

It was early in the morning when the nurse came in the room. Smiling, she asked, 'Are you ready?'

My answer was, 'As ready as possible. Let's get this over and done with!'

Then, the nurse gave me a tablet that would increase the strength of the anaesthesia. About thirty minutes after the tablet, I got an injection. By then I was half awake. A few minutes later, a doctor came to take me to theatre. My parents were sent to the waiting room and the operation started. I was already in theatre and the surgery was underway when Dr Angel arrived. As he entered the waiting room, he greeted my parents and patted my mother on the shoulder saying, 'Hang in there!'

When he left the waiting room, which was the entrance to the neurosurgery ward, my mother started freaking out. 'What is he doing here? Isn't he supposed to be in theatre? He said he would operate! Who is operating on my daughter?'

She tried to follow Dr Angel to ask what was going on, but my dad managed to prevent her. 'Don't complicate things. We do not know the whole story. Calm down.

It is a good thing Dad managed to stop her, because later they learnt that Dr Angel did not participate in the whole operation. Different people worked on different stages. He had a team of neurosurgeons. In my case, his team did the preparation – administering the anaesthesia, cutting my hair where the incision was going to be, opening the area just underneath the line of the skull for the extraction of the tumour. After all of that is done, Dr Angel performs. His only job was to extract the tumour. *Get all of it out!*

After many hours – roughly eight and a half – my parents saw Dr Angel come out of theatre. He went to his office. My parents saw him through the glass door between the entrance of the neu-rosurgery ward waiting room and the actual ward where all the patient rooms, theatres, doctors' offices were. A nurse followed, heading to the waiting room, and asked Mum and Dad to go to Dr Angel's office. As they walked, horrific thoughts plagued them. *What will he say? Why did it last so long? Did he remove all of the tumour?* He was still wearing his scrubs and looked awful. It was like someone had stolen ten years of his life. Normally, he was a handsome and appealing man but then he looked terrible.

When Mum and Dad were seated, he started. 'It was an exceedingly difficult operation. The tumour was big – the size of an orange. The whole thing is out. It looked like a ball, which meant that it had not metastasized. The battle is on her now. We did everything we could. Now it is her turn. She is currently in intensive care, hooked up to different devices for breathing, to monitor the heart, the bladder. The next twenty-four hours are critical. You cannot see her today, but I will arrange for you to see her on Saturday, that is tomorrow. You can go home because there's nothing you can do for her at this stage.'

After a pause he added, 'I am going to send Tihana to a reha-bilitation centre. It will be beneficial for her to start exercising immediately so that her muscles do not lose their strength com-pletely. There is a queue to get in, so I will reserve a spot now. Tihana will also need radiotherapy and chemotherapy after her rehabilitation. Because you live in Osijek, we will do it there, so you do not have to commute. I will write all the details about the radiotherapy – exactly where, the angle, the duration – and give them to our oncologist. He visits Osijek regularly, so in a month's time he will go and give the oncology ward in Osijek the instructions. It's not basic radiotherapy, so the oncologists need to know what to do and for how long.'

My parents spent the rest of the day praying in the hospital chapel. They were living in a hotel that was close to the hospital. Every two or three hours they called for information on my condition, and every time the answer was 'unchanged'.

Nothing in the world causes so much misery as uncertainty.[13]

'Unchanged' meant that in the first five hours after the operation I was completely unconscious. Later, I came to and was lingering between consciousness and unconsciousness, but more in the unconscious state. When I was conscious, I was aware of everyone and everything close to me but had no awareness of anything beyond the two-metre bubble around me. Anything beyond that bubble did not exist! It can be explained with the present moment. You know how they say that people must be in the present moment, and not in the past or the future? In that time, I could only be in the present moment. It was not possible (mentally) to be elsewhere. It was like someone limited me, and took away my thinking, perception, feeling and emotions. Basically, ninety-five percent of my mental abilities were gone. The remaining five percent served for understanding very plain things and comprehending what I saw with my limited eyesight. Apart from this, I could not speak.

There is a range of speech difficulties that can occur because of a brain tumour. The nature of the speech difficulty will depend upon the type, size and location of the tumour. I think I could not talk because my tumour had been in the left hemisphere, where most of the parts of the brain that control language are.

---

[13] Martin Luther; German professor of theology, composer, priest, Augustinian monk and seminal figure in the Protestant Reformation.

15

Intensive Care Unit

◇

The man who moves a mountain begins
by carrying away small stones.

~**Confucius**

On Saturday, the day after the operation, my parents arrived at the hospital to see me for the first time after the surgery. My state was the same, in that limbo where I was in between consciousness and unconsciousness. I do not know how to describe that. It was a weird thing, completely awkward! All I know is that one moment I was awake and understood everything I was told, but could not open my eyes nor speak, and had limited awareness. By limited awareness, I mean that I could comprehend everyone around me and understand why I was in the hospital, but that was it. And maybe thirty minutes or an hour later, I was out, not aware of anything. Totally unexplainable! I am assuming it has to do with the process of brain recovery.

From what I have learnt, recovery from brain surgery can take from four to eight weeks. The incisions may be sore for about five days after surgery. My incision was in between my ears, vertical and twelve cm long. I think it needed fifteen stiches or staples, which are usually taken out about one week after surgery, depending on the progress of recovery. The incision was on the back of my head. It stretched from the middle of my head to the end of my hairline. It was not thick, just a thin long line. And the doctors did not touch my scalp. Thank heavens for that! If they did it would have created additional issues. Dr Angel told Mum that cutting the scalp causes epilepsy, I guess because of connection it has with the nerves and blood. So, it was an exceptionally good thing that everything could be extracted without cutting my scalp.

Back to my parents... As they were approaching the intensive care unit, they were stopped by the main doctor there. My mum said, 'I'm the mother of Tihana Babic. She was operated on Friday. We have come to see her. Dr Angel allowed it.'

The doctor answered, 'Yes, I know that patient. That operation was extremely hard and dangerous. I am afraid I cannot authorise you to see her because of the danger you could impose on her. Do not worry, she is stable and recovering nicely, but unfortunately, I cannot allow you to see her. I do not understand how Dr Angel could have given you permission for that in the first place.'

They had a little dispute, but eventually the doctor caved. My parents think that she allowed it in the end because they were both so miserable and they basically pleaded.

When they entered the room, I was the only patient there, which could also be one of the reasons the doctor let them in. There were three more beds and mine was at the end of the room by the nurses' desk. I was covered with a sheet and my eyes were closed.

A million tubes were connected to me. I could hear everything they were saying but I could not open my eyes. Tears streamed down my face even though my eyes were shut. Even now, I do not understand how that is possible. I managed to mumble the word 'operation' just to let them know I could hear them and understand everything. They realised I was conscious. A huge relief for them. After that, I think I went into that limbo state because I cannot remember anything else.

Days slowly passed. My state was basically the same; the only difference was that after two days my conscious state lasted much longer, and I could partially open my eyes. Some days later, the doctors removed most of the tubes until only two were left, one for my lungs and another for my bladder. The reason I was in intensive care for so long was because my lungs were not working properly. They could not release me from intensive care until I could breathe on my own. Only then could I go to a normal hospital room.

During this time, my parents called repeatedly so they knew everything. They were just waiting to see me again. That would happen once the doctors allowed me to transfer to a normal room.

After ten days in the intensive care unit, my lungs recovered, and I could fully open my eyes. But I still could not go to my own room yet because they had to monitor my lungs. Though I was conscious and aware of where I was and why, it was a limited awareness. I was not in the position to form a whole, coherent sentence although I understood what others said. I did not think at that time probably because I could not. Basically, my state could be described as like an infant's; the only difference was that I understood some things and what people were saying.

On the thirteenth day in intensive care, I became more aware of my surroundings. I even began 'talking' – mainly repeating what someone would tell me. It was still impossible for me to form coherent sentences. At that point, my talking consisted of repeating what others said.

The reality was that I did not regain my old senses one hundred percent even long after the operation. I was aware of things more and more as time passed, but never in that stage was I completely aware. Hence, the talking issue was not a big deal for me. I cannot say it was ignorance. I just did not have the brain that would make me think that not speaking was a problem. This may seem stupid, but it felt like I was waking up and never getting to the stage of being fully awake. To make it a little more understandable, when I woke from the operation, I was in the state of an infant. As days passed in the hospital room, I 'grew' into a toddler, then into a child of ten years old, and then into an older child. But until 2015, I did not completely grow up. Well, sometimes I still think I have not entered the grown-up world. It is incomprehensible, but it did happen.

After fourteen days in the intensive care unit, I was finally released and transferred into a normal hospital room. My overall state was better, but I needed to adapt. Gradually move on, try to work with what was left after the surgery. Metaphorically speaking, the process was like building a house – and adding additional levels before checking whether the concrete foundations have set.

16

Aftermath Modification

Progress is not an illusion, it happens, but it is slow and invariably disappointing.

~George Orwell

When I arrived in my own room, there was some adapting to do. The people and surroundings made me feel like a child that had just left the security of their mother's womb. It was a juvenile feeling, which was not in accordance with my age, but that is the accurate term to describe that feeling. In the intensive care unit, I was dealing with one, maybe two people, tops. But in the hospital room, it was a completely different story. My roomies left, so I got new ones, new nurses and new doctors.

Thankfully, my parents were always by my side. They were only absent during the night. The nurses were not necessary because Mum and Dad did almost everything for me. My parents put their lives on hold to do so. They left everything to look after me. Talk about sacrifice! Those people – Mirela and Zvonimir – are two true angels walking on Earth.

I still had a catheter because I was not allowed to stand yet, but that did not last for long. As I recall, after a day, the doctor told me that it is was beneficial to start moving. Something about blood flow and muscles. It was impossible to walk on my own. My parents would hold me, one on each side, and we would go to the toilet and take little walks down the corridor. And by walk, I mean basically being held upright by my parents.

My brain sustained injuries to the motor cortex. That is the part of the brain involved in planning, controlling and executing voluntary movements. In my case, everything I once had was altered or lost. Mostly lost.

The tumour was located on the left side of my brain, so the right side of the body was affected. The use of my right hand was non-existent. The left one was not so good either. My right leg was not participating at all. The left leg helped, but only so much. I could not go to the toilet on my own, let alone wash myself. I had difficulty swallowing. It took me forty-five minutes to eat a small yogurt. I could not feed myself or hold a cup of water, so my mum and dad fed me and gave me beverages. I still could not form a sentence. I would just repeat things others would say. I think that changed after I got out of the hospital when I went to rehabilitation.

Eventually the stitches in my head had to be removed. They were not removed as they usually are, five days after the surgery. Mine were in for lot longer, a total of eighteen days. Although it was a big cut, having the stitches out did not hurt – maybe just a sting here and there.

With time, my whole body, inside and out, was slowly healing. I think, my body was completely shaken up by the operation and some things ended up in places they should not be in. Like an earthquake, everything needed time to be repaired and put back in the right place. Every day that passed meant more progress. Everything in my body was working simultaneously and in conjunction with one another to progress. Slowly, I was becoming my old self, re-entering my life.

As time passed, my motor control issues changed because the tumour affected my cerebellum or 'hindbrain'. It is the region of the brain that plays an important role in motor control. The cerebellum does not initiate movement, but contributes to coordination, and the precision and timing of movements. Cerebellar damage produces disorders in fine movement, equilibrium, posture and motor learning.

I was diagnosed with ataxia. Ataxia is a lack of muscle control or coordination for voluntary movements, such as walking or picking up objects. A sign of an underlying condition, ataxia can affect various movements, and create difficulties with speech, eye movement and swallowing. It was dreadful knowing that a simple task like touching my nose with my right hand was mission impossible at first. All those impairments were a lot more troubling once I got home, to the point that even now, years later, I need to keep exercising. There were many issues, some of which have diminished or vanished over time.

Physically, some of my problems included a lack of control especially over the right side of my body. At first it was not possible to do any aimed or precise movements. I could not walk on my own. Writing was impossible with my right hand. My speech was at the level of a toddler's, repeating the words others said. There were many other issues. My vision in my right eye was affected. My hearing in the right ear was diminished. I had trouble swallowing and as a result had extensive saliva. Must I go on?

On the appearance side, I needed electrotherapy for my face. Electrotherapy is the use of electrical energy as a medical treatment. In medicine, the term electrotherapy can apply to a variety of treatments, including the use of electrical devices such as deep brain stimulators for neurological diseases. In my case, the muscles on the right side of my face had completely weakened causing the right side of my face to droop. We used to joke that my face resembled our former president's face. Everyone, including me, made fun of him when we saw him in the paper or on television. I am not sure what the exact amount of electrotherapy needed was, but after fifteen to twenty sessions, lasting fifteen to twenty minutes, my face returned to normal. Thankfully, my voice was not affected so much, but it was still a bit altered. I spoke slower than usual, but other than that everything was fine.

I stayed in hospital for twenty-one days after the operation. When they discharged me, a wonderful emotion came over me. It is a pity I could not jump, because I wanted to. I remembered a commercial for Toyota. Without the jumping part, the words, 'Oh, what a feeling!' sprang from my lips. After twenty-one days inside a building with no sun, no fresh air, nothing, the sunshine felt incredible. I was happy just breathing the air, seeing the surroundings. Being in the hospital made me feel as if life had stopped. Everything outside had been frozen all that time, as if I had paused my favourite soap opera and returned after a month at the exact same spot. Nothing had changed. Some things had changed but life indeed moves on. Relentlessly!

17

Rehabilitation Centre

◇

*Do what you must do, until you can do
what you want to do.*

~Oprah Winfrey

*D*r Angel told my parents that right after my discharge from the hospital, I would be sent to a rehabilitation centre. All the patients from Rebro Hospital were sent to a rehabilitation centre in Krapina. It is the best rehabilitation centre in Croatia in terms of facilities, results, equipment and different types of hydrotherapy. It focused on post-operative patients.

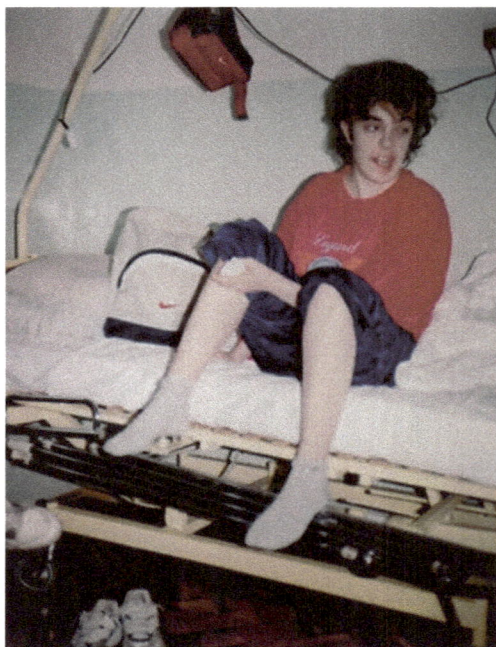

Krapina Rehabilitation Centre post-operation

The town of Krapina is in the middle of a region called Zagorje in north-western Croatia. A river called Krapinčica flows through the town. The town's name is tightly linked to that river. Specifically, the Krapinčica river is full of carp, known as 'krap' in the local Kajkavian dialect. Hence, the name Krapina. It was a genuinely nice place. The surroundings were calm, green, peaceful and beautiful. The river enriched the town to the degree that it appeared to be more of a holiday retreat than a rehabilitation centre, somewhere to escape life's routine. A place where you can let yourself go and unwind. Krapina is a well-known historical town, most famous for the discovery of Neanderthal skeletons there in 1899 – Krapinian Early Man.

The rehabilitation centre in Krapina was equipped with all sorts of devices. There was a special area reserved for hydrotherapy. There were so many different specific therapies: cardio therapy, work therapy[14], speech therapy, electrotherapy. The staff explained that it was less a hospital, and more a place equipped for physiotherapy and recreation. People there had the opportunity to go out and enjoy the sun and scenery. That way exercise did not seem so boring.

My room was okay. The only issue was that it was so dark, the light needed to be on most of the time. Even though it was a hospital, it did not seem like one. It was very uplifting and without that hospital smell. I was lucky that I was mobile. When I say mobile, I mean I wasn't in a wheelchair. I can say that I did walk a bit better when I left the hospital, but still my parents stood on either side of me. At least I was leaning more on my legs. Every now and then, my parents would take me out for coffee and a cake, something else that made it feel more like a spa than a hospital.

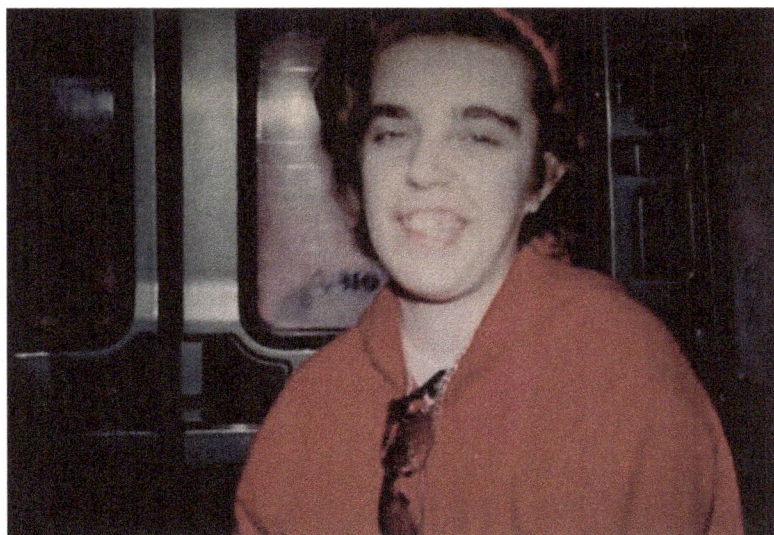

In Krapina – Mixing business with pleasure

---

[14] Work therapy, also known as occupational therapy, is a broad term covering interventions designed to facilitate someone's return to work after an injury or illness.

After I got settled in, a doctor and a speech therapist came to sort out my schedule. As they were working it out, they began arguing. Slowly, it turned into a shouting match. The appropriate words for this squabble would be *childish competition*. You know when two five-year-olds fight over whose toys are better? These two were disputing who was better and whose medical field was more useful. The power of vanity among doctors! My dad flipped out and said, 'If you two don't quit it immediately, I will put this in the newspaper. My daughter came out of an extremely hard operation and needs rest. She's not here to listen to your nonsense!' After my dad's words, they both calmed down and were as smooth as butter – nice, polite, in whatever-you-want-or-need mode. Sometimes showing your teeth does the trick.

My schedule turned out to be packed with different exercises: electrotherapy, speech therapy, hydrotherapy massage, work therapy and physiotherapy. All of these were badly needed so I couldn't say no to any one of them. The electrotherapy was for my face. The doctors told me that it would be beneficial to have it twice a week. As I have noted in the previous chapter, my voice and speech did not change very much, but nonetheless weekly speech therapy was scheduled. I don't know why, but I did not argue. Hydrotherapy massage, which is water massage, was needed to wake up my muscles, so it was scheduled for three times a week. My work therapy included different hand exercises that I needed to improve my motor skills and their precision. This was scheduled for three times a week too. And the icing on the cake – physiotherapy. Five times a week. I had a lot on my plate but no complaints. I had no time for self-pity or negativity.

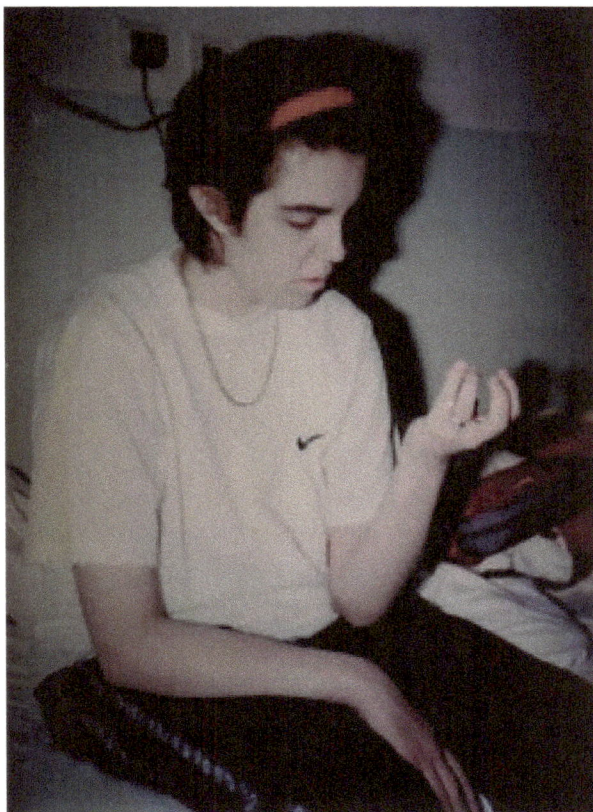

Living with the aftermath

My parents were with me all the time, except at night. They took me to my different therapies and outside. Aside from all my blessings, this was another incredibly significant one for me. Aside from exercises and outings, I also got to spend time with familiar faces – my parents. Thank God that they were able to do all that financially and the fact that they put their lives on hold for me meant a lot. I do not know how to repay them for their constant love, care, understanding, faith – the list goes on. Love is paid with love.

My ability to wash myself, feed myself, go to the toilet and generally take care of my body was non-existent. Someone had to help me at all times in the beginning. As time passed, the need for help diminished, but it was never entirely absent. Looking back, I would say that those days after the operation and my stay in Krapina were the most challenging. Later, everything was a tiny bit easier, but an even bigger challenge awaited – going home and adapting.

Even though I was not one hundred percent aware and sane, some things were apparent and could not be ignored. I knew who I was, where I was, what happened, why I was in Krapina and what I was doing there. But I was not completely lucid. It can be best explained with a comparison to alcohol: after drinking quite a lot, a person is kind of numb and everything is a bit clouded in their head. That was my state of mind for two or three months after my tumour was removed, but, as I noted before, it took even longer to completely regain my consciousness. At that time, my awareness was based on the fact that I needed help, that someone needed to feed me, wash me, take me to the toilet. I was an infant aged eighteen. I could have passed as a cute baby girl if only my body wasn't so big. Shame!

18

Reconstruction

Sometimes we survive by forgetting.

–Unknown

As time passed, things were slowly progressing. My whole physical state improved but the psychological side effects started showing. This happened due to the slow recovery of my brain. Negative and destructive thoughts started appearing, but they were not frequent, and thankfully because of my busy schedule, I did not have the time to address them properly. My schedule was so tight that I barely had any free time, mainly because of physiotherapy and work therapy. Other than that, I quite enjoyed hydrotherapy massage, and going out for coffee and cake. But, with time, the thoughts started piling up and I could no longer control them. They were extremely negative, so much so that even I was afraid of the things that popped into my head. For that reason, I started to see a psychologist in order to revise my thoughts thoroughly. At times, I felt like those filthy rich people who have their own therapist to whom they can spill their guts. It was cool to have your own person to whine and pine to!

Throughout my stay there, I was working with an incredibly good physiotherapist. At first my enthusiasm towards her was rather poor. Everyone there said she was extremely strict and particular about her work. Physiotherapy must be done correctly. There is no other way for it. If you want good results, aside from your own motivation and will, your therapist must be persistent with heaps of knowledge and skill. That approach helped a lot. The first couple of hours with her were not so promising. But seeing that her methods were effective, my attitude changed to the point that I enjoyed exercising with her and looked forward to it. Apart from being thrilled with her results, I must admit I was intimidated by her. I had to follow her instructions to the letter, especially when she was watching. I have had poor posture all my life, and that became even worse after the operation. So, our exercising goal was to improve my posture among other things.

I remember one episode with her. It felt so embarrassing, but I still laughed like crazy. My parents and I were going out for coffee and cake. My parents were walking beside me just in case I fell. My posture was, as usual, hunched, as it was when nobody corrected me. I was ignoring my physiotherapist's instructions and doing my kind of walking. In the rehab centre, there were four hallways that were all connected in a circle. From my room on the first floor, we had to pass two hallways to get to the lift. The first hallway was okay, and the second started off the same way. But just as we approached the lift, my physio spotted me. I think the whole institution heard her yell, 'Tihana, straighten up!' Immediately, I lifted my upper body. It was such a quick reaction that my parents started laughing. It was like when a teacher walks in a classroom – sudden obedience. We still laugh when we remember that.

Despite the reason for my being there, I generally enjoyed rehab. I was in a beautiful place, getting stronger every day. But it was not all smooth sailing.

When word about my diagnosis spread to my close friends and neighbourhood, everyone started to drift away. Then and there, I found out who was with me through thick and thin, and who was a fair-weather friend. It was not just friends and acquaintances, but even some relatives too. Maybe they did not know how to handle the situation, or how to handle me. Either way, it hurt. I do not have a grudge towards these people, nor hold on to bad memories about feeling abandoned. Still, feelings of resentment or anger towards some people are present. Maybe my ego is huge, but some people's actions and reactions changed my perspective towards them. They lost their place on my personal value list. You can repair a building after an earthquake, but it will never be the same building. My relationships with some people were damaged beyond repair. This sounds harsh, I know, but some things simply cannot be forgotten. I have issues forgiving myself, let alone someone else.

One person amazed me. Her name is Marija and she is about my age. Her grandparents lived across the street from my house, so we would play together every time she visited them. I had known her for as long as I can remember. It was not a day-to-day friendship, but we understood each other and had the same views on some things. During my stay in Krapina, she called me every single night for twenty-one days, talking to me as if I was a normal person. She was not afraid or uncomfortable with me at all. On the contrary, she accepted me for who I was, regardless of what had happened. That struck a chord in my heart. Out of all the people who abandoned me, she emerged to be a true friend and someone I could rely on besides my parents. *A real friend is one who walks in when the rest of the world walks out.* We still are good friends, and she will always have a special place in my heart. The fact that she embraced me and my situation without holding back at all speaks volumes and shows the true meaning of friendship.

19

Homecoming

◇

In three words I can sum up everything I've learned
about life: it goes on.

~Robert Frost

t the end of April 2003, I left the rehabilitation centre in Krapina and returned home. Finally, after exactly fifty-one days, I was back on known soil, in a familiar place. Spring was ongoing, and the weather was perfect. Sunny clear blue skies, just ideal. We had a large backyard, which I enjoyed quite a bit. It let me be out in the sun breathing in the fresh air. As our house was on the corner of the street, the backyard extended around three sides of our house. The area in front of the house faced a park. All was filled with greenery, tranquillity and relaxation. On the second side, the backyard was very spacious, and faced the street and other houses. We had two driveways for the two garages. The third section of the backyard had a lawn and the pool. The pool was not in use because it needed repairing, but that did not worry me. I was not a big pool lover anyway.

I did all kinds of things – exercise, walk, work therapy, relax and enjoy the scenery, read. Being home meant easygoing, relaxed rehabilitation. Well, easygoing in some ways –my radiation and chemotherapy awaited.

Physically, I still needed a little help in doing the activities of daily life – washing myself, going to the toilet – but I got a wheelchair, which made life easier. I made slow progress in my exercises and other therapies, but progress, nonetheless. Eventually, I could wash my face, brush my teeth and go to the toilet on my own. But I was still only semi-able in the shower and had issues with some other things like tying my shoes or buttoning something up.

On a less pleasant note, I had to have an MRI of my head and spine every six months in the beginning. This was to monitor my condition, check for a recurrence or other issues. A year after the operation, the frequency was reduced to annually. But even now, I am not at all pleased when the MRI is due. Currently, the scan is scheduled for every three years. Out of all the tests I've had, this one is the most boring. It's extremely dull. The process involves lying completely still for fifty minutes in a tube only sixty centimetres wide. I mean the tube is sixty centimetres in width and in depth. So, you cannot completely relax, nor move a lot. Topping off this wonderful event, they include an injection of contrast agents. The contrast agents are necessary to discover any changes in the scans, but it is not a nice thing to be poked. I have had more than enough needles. *Extreme dislike!* Every now and then, I have an additional scan that lasts twenty minutes. This one is done as a precaution because my type of tumour usually spreads to the head area and the spine.

To prevent a relapse, I took heaps of natural products – vitamins, minerals, antioxidants, immune system supports. I have tried them all, old and new natural medicines. Out of the whole variety of herbs and vitamins, some were useful, some less so. At first, I was using CaliVita products. I took vitamin C, vitamin A, B complex vitamins, vitamin D, Selenium. This information is particularly important, so I believe it should be attended to solemnly. One whole chapter will be dedicated to this topic because I think that this information could be useful for other people in similar situations.

Psychologically, everything seemed to be in order at first, but as time went by, negative and destructive thoughts surfaced. Thoughts like *the tumour will come back. I will never get rid of it. My destiny is this wheelchair. My leg will be amputated.* Some of these negative thoughts had roots in reality, but some were irrational and in no way could be a possible outcome given my diagnosis. But I was terrified, so that is my excuse. I even blamed and cursed God for my misfortune.

My questions at that time, which do not differ all that much now, were what did I do to deserve this punishment? My actions as a child and teenager did not surpass the boundaries of normal behaviour. School-wise, everything was in control. I was an A-grade student, did all my assignments, did not skip lessons. Socially, I was not outgoing as it were, but I did not drink nor smoke, or God forbid, do drugs. Basically, I went by all the rules, never bending them on any terms. All of that made me think, *how does someone who does everything by the book get punished like this, while some people do terrible things to their health, and they are completely fine.* It is not fair! Usually if people play with fire eventually, they get burned. I get that, but what I cannot understand is, why do people who do not play with fire not only get burned, but fully blazed? That really infuriates me! *I know there is no rea-sonable answer. But still, why?* These dark thoughts plagued me to the point that I needed to seek professional help. The worst bullies you will ever encounter in your life are your own thoughts.[15]

Since my family is packed with doctors, once again Mum con-tacted her cousin's wife, the gynaecologist, to ask her if she knew a good psychiatrist. She remembered a friend of hers from university. She was exceptionally good at what she does and very professional. I started to have regular sessions with her at the end of 2003. Instead of doing plain psychiatry work, she was my psychologist also.

Psychiatrists are specialised medical doctors who can diagnose illness, manage treatment, and provide a range of therapies for complex and serious mental illness. They have the power to pre-scribe medications. Psychologists are not doctors. They cannot pre-scribe medication or diagnose illnesses. Instead, psychologists focus on providing psychotherapy (talking therapy) to help patients. I was lucky to have a psychiatrist and psychologist all in one.

We discussed so many things and she really helped lighten the situation. Because my state of mind was very dark, depres-sion was slowly but surely consuming me. Very soon after meeting me, she told my mum and me that because my head had been opened during the operation to remove my tumour, my brain experienced a shock that caused an interruption in the secretion of serotonin. Serotonin is a neurotransmitter that regulates mus-cle contraction, body temperature, pain, appetite, mood swings, blood pressure and breathing. Not having that neurotransmitter explains everything. The reason for those dark negative thoughts, for that depression I was in, was serotonin. In order to re-establish the secretion of this neurotransmitter, she prescribed me a drug

---

[15] Bryant McGill, an American author, activist and social entrepreneur.

called Fevarin that is meant to improve mental health and your emotional condition. She said, 'I don't want to give you anything stronger because I believe it's just a matter of re-establishing secretion. The dosage will be half a tablet, which is fifty milligrams daily. This amount is not addictive. My aim is for the drug to get the ball rolling and then you can slowly come off it.'

The medication helped very much. Not long after I started taking it, the dark thoughts were diminishing and my mood in general was better.

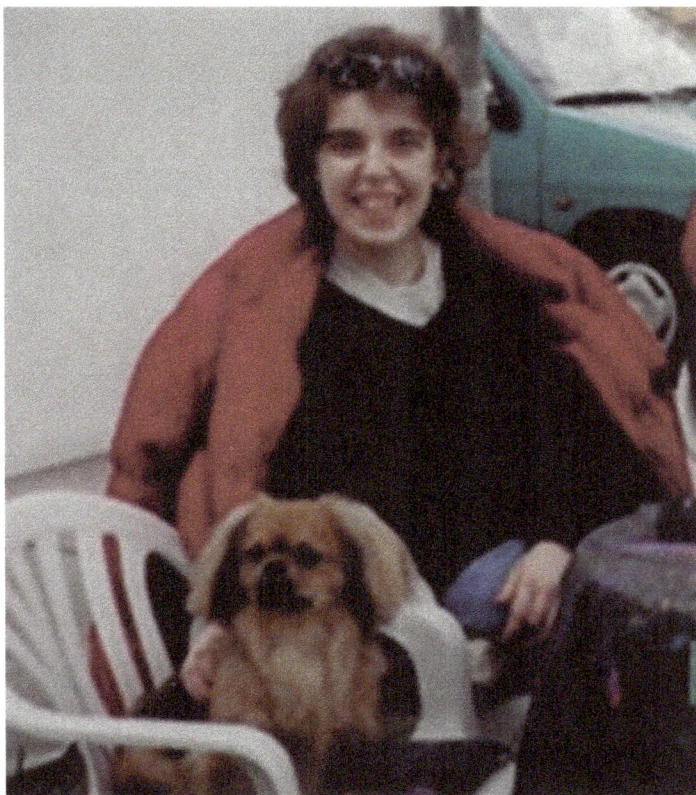

After the first operation - reassembled me

It took maybe a year for everything to fall into place. I made slower progress with walking and work therapy than with the mental health issues. I think that, in general, recuperating was 'easier' because one side of my body was intact. As we know, the brain is divided into two hemispheres, the left and the right. These two hemispheres can function together or individually. Because the brain is cross-networked, damage in one side of the brain hits the opposite side of the body. In my case, the damage was on the left side of the brain, which meant that the right side of my body was affected. So, the right side of my body (the damaged side) could 'lean on' the left side (the intact side). This made rehabilitation much faster and I was able to walk shortly after my stay in Krapina. My walking could not be described as perfect, but it was quick. I made mistakes, especially when I started walking, but the mistakes lessened as I got used to walking. As I progressed, my gait got better but remained fast. Later, my physiotherapist told me that the speed was caused by momentum. He said it was a physics thing. Another name for it is mass in motion. Basically, the greater the momentum, the faster the walk. If I walk fast, I walk better with fewer mistakes. That is the way I understood his words.

The ability to have a more homely, relaxed rehabilitation was refreshing. It was easygoing without stress and scheduled sessions. On the flip side of the coin, that kind of rehabilitation gives you more room for skulking. And I must say that sometimes I overused that privilege.

20

Radiation and Chemotherapy

Without patient endurance even, the smallest thing becomes unbearable. A lot depends on our attitude.

~Dalai Lama

This chapter covers my radiotherapy and chemotherapy, what it meant and how I felt.

Radiation therapy or radiotherapy, often abbreviated to RT, RTx or XRT, is a therapy using ionizing radiation. It is generally used as part of cancer treatment to control or kill malignant cells. Radiation therapy is commonly used to treat cancerous tumours because of its ability to moderate cell growth. Ionizing radiation works by damaging the DNA of cancerous tissue leading to cellular death.

While I was recuperating from the operation in Rebro, my parents sorted out my radiation and chemotherapy. Or rather, Dr Angel arranged everything. An oncologist from Rebro would give instructions to the oncologist in Osijek. These directions were necessary since I would not be having basic radiation therapy. I do not know how my radiotherapy differed from normal. My assumption is that maybe the radiation was not directed at my whole head, just on the part where the tumour was. There are two reasons for this thought. One, there was no need for radiation on my whole head; the tumour had not metastasized elsewhere. Two, Rebro Hospital is innovative, and embraces doing things out of the ordinary and introducing new ideas. That may be a logical explanation for the difference, but I do not know the real cause for my special treatment.

Anyway, a couple of days after our return home from Krapina, we got called in to Osijek Hospital. I was introduced to my radiation oncologist and a meeting took place. He told me everything had been scheduled and set up for the radiation process to start. I had been given an informed consent form to sign. During that meeting, I found out how the radiotherapy would be performed, how long the procedure would last and how many sessions I would need. I was having external beam radiation therapy, which delivers radiation from a machine outside of the body. This type of radiation therapy targets only the tumour. That said, inevitably, it will affect some neighbouring healthy tissue. The healthy cells around where the tumour was are able to regenerate themselves, but the cancerous cells can't. Each session would be quick and painless, lasting about fifteen minutes. I would have to go five times per week, Monday through to Friday. The two-day pause – Saturday and Sunday – in treatment each week was to give my body a chance to repair and prepare for the next lot. This would be my life for the next two months. At the end of the meeting, the doctor said that they – the oncologists – needed to make a thermoplastic mask for my head. The purpose of this mask is to secure my head so that the radiation beams would be directed in the right spot. It is a mesh mask, moulded to my face and secured to the table. It took a couple of days for the doctors to adjust the radiation – find the right angle, the correct pathway, the exact location of the removed tumour – and make the mask. After that, radiation commenced. It was not painful or uncomfortable. The peculiar thing with me is that my hair did not fall out, unlike in almost all cases. Seems I really am in the one percent!

The radiation finally ended. It was not hard or troubling, nor did it hurt. On the contrary, it was quite pleasant. Obviously, the scenario was not good at all, but throughout the procedure you could lie down and relax. I did not have to do anything. As soon as my radiation was completed, chemotherapy awaited.

After all the mistreatment and heartache, the doctors in Osijek Hospital had caused me, I was amazed how they followed Dr Angel's instructions to the letter. I was expecting resistance from them about being told what to do by someone else. I cannot forget my earlier encounters with doctors. Everything that happened was exhausting and incredibly sad. Nowadays, when I hear the word 'doctor', ill will consumes me. I know I have issues with certain things, but it is hard for me to ignore that those things happened. If I could only embrace my past and turn to the present and future. Every time I try, something happens that make me remember. *The past cannot be changed, forgotten, edited or erased; it can only be accepted.*

Chemotherapy – chemo – is medicine used to weaken and destroy cancer cells in the body, including cells at the original cancer site and any that may have spread to another part of the body (metastasized). It is a systemic therapy, which means it affects the whole body by going through the bloodstream.

My type of tumour required a certain chemotherapy that highly differs from the conventional way of doing it, a drip infused into a vein. Again, the reason why is unknown to me. Nevertheless, the doctors made up a schedule for me based on the instructions they had been given by Zagreb. My schedule comprised of six cycles. After each cycle, I would have a blood test. This was to ensure the numbers of erythrocytes (red blood cells), leukocytes (white blood cells) and thrombocytes (platelets) were normal. They must not be too high or too low. Each cycle lasted about a month and consisted of three steps.

Firstly, I took two tablets and waited ten days for the tablets to do their thing. Secondly, I had an injection and twenty days later came the third and final step – another injection. To make everything clear, I do not know what the tablets did and if their effect was long lasting. I am sure that both injections were the same, but again their impact is unknown. Everything was explained to me prior, but that particular information was not important to me.

As I noted, my blood was checked after every cycle of chemotherapy. My blood cell levels were normal for three cycles, but after the fourth they begun to drop drastically. I made it through the fourth cycle but could not continue. All my blood cell numbers had plunged, but especially the erythrocytes. That was extremely dangerous, so my radiologist said we should stop the chemotherapy. There were many risks, but my doctor was worried about three things in particular: infection, anaemia, and bleeding and bruising. Infection was extra likely because a low level of leukocytes means that your body is less able to fight off infection. That is why a blood cell level plunge is an emergency if you're having chemotherapy. Anaemia is dangerous because chemotherapy drugs can lower the number of erythrocytes in the blood, leaving you tired, weak, faint and short of breath. Bleeding and bruising were a risk because chemotherapy can lower the number of thrombocytes in your blood, leading to a condition called thrombocytopenia. If the number of platelets drops, you may be more likely to have nosebleeds, bleeding gums or tiny red spots on your skin. You may also bruise more easily than normal.

Generally, I did not feel pain after the treatment. That is on the physical side. Psychologically, it was a totally different story. After the second cycle, I was in an awfully bad state and from there my mental health kept deteriorating. I was plagued by dark thoughts of disaster, calamity, tragedy, death. *Unbelievably bad!* At the end of the recovery period between each cycle, I would come to my old self again, and then – bang! – another cycle would start. When I heard we were going to stop, on the one hand I was relieved. Those thoughts were hard to get through. But on the other, I was in a panic. *Are four cycles enough? What if?* I had a million what ifs, and for every single one, there was a worse ending. *Bad, worse, worst!*

21

Natural Alleviation

◇

Nature itself is the best physician.

~**Hippocrates**

*I*n this chapter about remedies and vitamins, I explain measures I took during my recovery, along with information and my evaluation of their effectiveness.

Before I get into everything, I want to note that the solemn reason for all this – the natural remedies, vitamins and self-help – is my mother. When we arrived home from Krapina, Mum started investigating all-natural remedies and things that are beneficial for different conditions and illnesses. In her investigations, she found that acid in the body is a possible risk factor in developing cancer. Cancer cells differ from normal cells in the body in many ways. Normal cells become cancerous when a series of mutations leads the cell to continue to grow and divide out of control. In a way, a cancer cell is a cell that has achieved a sort of immortality. An acidic environment favours the growth of cancer cells. It is best to stay around the middle of the pH scale – not too acidic and not too basic. Like everything in life, aim to achieve the golden middle.

Later, Mum discovered that inflammation in the body also causes cancer. Inflammation refers to your body's process of fighting against things that harm it, such as infections, injuries and toxins, in an attempt to heal itself. When something damages your cells, your body releases chemicals that trigger a response from your immune system.

My belief is that both pH and inflammation can be changed and modified by diet and supplements. The diet for these two things includes lots of green vegetables, some fruits and nuts. A pH scale can be found on the internet, but the basic instruction is to avoid dairy products and meat. Dairy products cause inflammation. Meat is acidic. Some people stick to this as their holy grail; I am not one of them. My thoughts are eat everything, but in moderation! I would be lying if I said that I do not monitor what I eat or drink, but I do not go to extremes. Sweet things like cakes, chocolate and fruit yogurts are acidic, but I cannot claim I do not eat them. My rule is to eat more of the good things and less of the bad things. Moderation, moderation, moderation!

My overall diet and beverages dramatically changed after my diagnosis. As I noted before, I was a keen meat eater, especially preserved meat, which is cancerous, and especially pork. I cannot say I did not eat it, nor can I say I don't consume it now. However, the amount has drastically reduced to no more than two to four slices per week, and there were weeks it was not consumed whatsoever. In general, my diet changed to the better, to be healthier.

My mum is one of those people who does not believe in tablets or medicine. From her point of view, tablets and medicine only fix the temporary problem but they do not kill the root. By not eliminating the root cause, the problem will come back. She has always believed that, as has my father. I never thought about it prior to my distressful event. Thankfully, I had not had any major health issues before that. My only problem was allergic asthma, so there had been minimal need for tablets or medicine. As a child I got it once I moved to Australia, and it has been present since then. Sometimes the attacks were severe to the point I had to go to the Emergency Room, but generally I would describe it as mild. I have my Ventolin and Seretide inhalers; that's all.

Living and coping with the aftermath of my brain tumour, I have started to believe in natural medicine, and agree with my parents that modern medicine does not destroy the root of the problem. Better put, I am positive conventional medicine does not eliminate the root of the problem. My issue is with strength: does natural medicine have enough power to battle difficult illnesses? My beliefs are not so strong yet. I am not completely convinced. Throughout my journey, it is evident that I only once rejected anything the doctors said or advised. Later, I explain why. My journey proves that natural medicine does indeed help.

In the first months after returning from Krapina, I started drinking all sorts of vitamins. These vitamins were used to prevent cancer. Vitamin C, along with magnesium, is vital for our bodies. It protects the body from bacteria and viruses. Vitamin A is important for normal vision, the immune system and reproduction. It helps the heart, lungs, kidneys and other organs work properly. B complex vitamins are needed for optimal health; they impact appetite, vision, the skin, nerves and red blood cell formation. Vitamin D is for the brain, nervous system and bones. Selenium – nutritionally essential for humans – is a constituent of more than two dozen selenoproteins that play critical roles in reproduction, thyroid hormone metabolism and DNA synthesis.

As if that weren't enough, selenium also offers protection from oxidative damage and infection. All these vitamins protect from cancer, but are not specifically listed in mainstream medicine. Mind you, I still consume them.

Basically, my belief is that cancer is not caused by only one thing. I think multiple factors contribute to its development and all the remedies I used help. My thoughts formed from my experience and the research I did after the whole cancer ordeal was stamped and sealed. It is said that three elements – body, mind and soul – should be in sync for our systems to maintain normal function and health. In my case, I was out of sync. Body-wise, I had a bad diet. There was lots acidity and inflammation, and I did not exercise. My mind whirled with bad and destructive thoughts. I felt anger and resentment towards anyone who did me wrong. My soul was heavy with emotions and feelings of sadness, negativity and stress. There you have it: for me, that is a certain recipe for illness or disorder in the body.

Aside from vitamins, I also took natural tablets called Culevit. The tablets are a mixture of vitamins and amino acids essential for regenerating and strengthening the body in cases of serious illnesses, diminished health, weight loss and general ill health. Some people refer to these tablets as natural chemotherapy. The tablets were taken hourly. I swallowed one tablet every hour, from eight o'clock in the morning to eight o'clock in the evening. This totalled thirteen tablets per day, for fourteen days, followed by a two-month break.

Searching for natural medicine that guards the body from cancer, Mum was online and crossed paths with a medicine that kills cancer cells. That medicine had a profound impact on me, to the point that I am still using it. I do not know if or when I am going to stop. This miracle cure is called the Budwig diet or the

Budwig protocol – an alternative treatment that can be utilized to complement traditional cancer therapy. It consists of linseed oil (also known as flaxseed oil) mixed with cottage cheese. Yogurt or kefir can be used instead of cottage cheese. These three – cottage cheese, yogurt, and kefir – are nothing but conductors. The reason for this is that linseed oil on its own is not absorbed into the body; a conductor is needed. Additionally, ground linseeds can be added, noting to consume the concoction within fifteen minutes of grinding, or else the linseeds lose their beneficial properties. Personally, I add linseeds because they are healthy. They contain omega-3 fatty acids, which are proven to have some effect on cancer cells. They reduce the levels of certain chemicals associated with cancer. Linseeds also contain substances called lignans and phytoestrogens that both have anti-cancer and hormonal effects. I do not care for official approval; I believe in it!

There is a liquid remedy my Aunt Ljerka told my mum about, called noni juice. She said that it is a beneficial anti-cancer natural medicine. There are a lot of different brands of noni juice. I used Tahitian and Polynesian noni juice. At that time, the word was that those two were the purest noni juices around. The juice consists of eighty-nine percent noni fruit, and eleven percent grape and blueberry juice concentrates. Out of its many benefits, the most important for me were anti-inflammatory properties, anti-cancer properties. It strengthens cell structure and boosts the immune system. It really has widespread benefits for lots of different illnesses. Plus, it tastes nice too. At first, I was drinking half a liter daily, then the dosage was reduced. All in all, I consumed it for nearly a year. After that I stopped. By the suggestions of people who make it and sell it, the juice had fulfilled its purpose.

Another remedy was sent by Mum's cousin Vlado in Serbia, Croatia's neighbour. Vlado had heard about my illness and wanted to help. Serbia had a well-known doctor who used to practise medicine in a military hospital in Banjica, Serbia. After some time, he decided to switch from official medicine to alternative medicine. He opened a cancer clinic that focused on healing cancer using natural medicine. Anyway, Vlado asked for all my medical documents so that the doctor there could make a proper health package for me. The package consisted of six big jars of herbs mixed with honey, and three big packs of detox tea. My diet was made up of the package he sent, combined with vegetables, fruit and nuts. No animal products – no meat, no dairy products, no eggs. A vegan diet. Vlado's regime was to last forty-two days.

My doctors were firmly against that kind of diet. They claimed that due to the upcoming radiotherapy and chemotherapy, my diet should be a broad variety of nutrients: meat, fish, diary, vegetables, eggs, fruit, and nuts. In their opinion, the body needed nourishment prior to and during radiotherapy and chemotherapy. We – my parents and I – decided to do it despite my doctors' advice. I knew it was a risk, but not having cancer was more important. *For the rest of my life I pledge that I will take anti-cancer actions, despite the risk!*

My belief is that every little thing I did was worth it. If nothing else, those remedies delayed the recurrence for six years.

22

Informal Rehabilitation

◇

A great step towards independence is a good-humoured stomach, one that is willing to endure rough treatment.

~Lucius Annaeus Seneca

As time passed, everything was improving by the day. Exercising and all the natural medicine I used really helped. I was doing everything independently by September 2004. Do not misinterpret my words, it was independent according to my new abilities. I was able to do everyday things like wash and feed myself, nothing complicated. I still could not do any detailed work with my hands. Work therapy did help with that – precisely touching something, tying and untying knots, practising doing buttons up. Even though I managed to do those things, everything was slower in comparison to before the operation. It took a lot of hard work, fury, frustration and tears, but I could do everything myself.

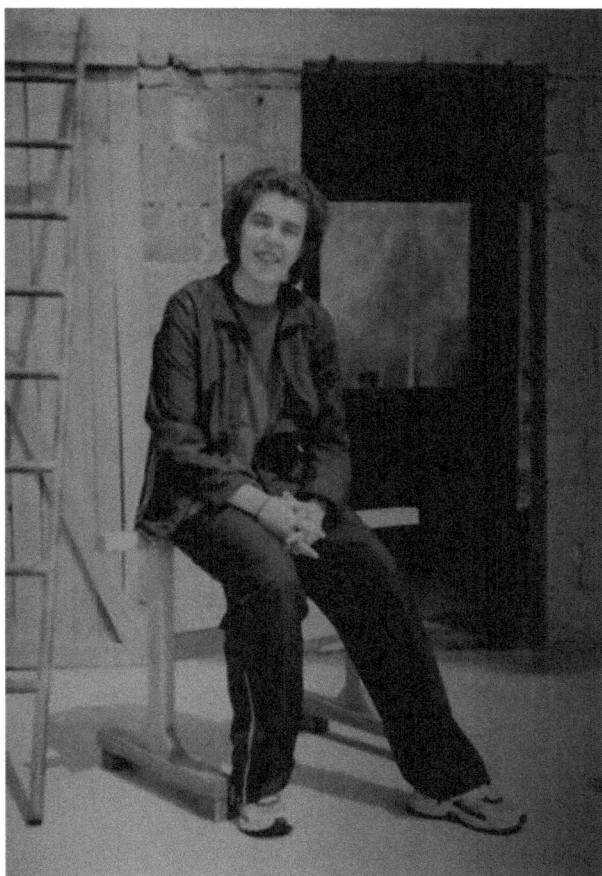

3 years afer the first operation

I could walk independently again, but my gait was faster than usual because of the momentum. Once I had picked up the gist of everyday walking again, there were no mistakes, just fast walking. I remember every time I would go for a walk with my parents, I was always two metres ahead. I just could not slow down. *But I was walking!*

As I noted previously, my Aunt Snježana was a great help in that department. Almost every day we would go walking. I just had to call her, and she would come in an instant, ready for anything. She could keep up with me, being a fast walker herself, and she loved walking. It was mainly long-distance walking, which was greatly beneficial for me. We would go to the centre of Osijek and watch the world go by or relax in parks. All that walking was rewarding for me after being in bed for a long time. I am so grateful to her. She sacrificed her private time for me. What a wonderful, selfless act. Thank you from the bottom of my heart! RIP.

My writing was still an issue. Usually I am right-handed, but due to the damage from the tumour, I learnt to write with my left hand. It was slow and it annoyed me. Repetition makes everything better; that is so clear to me. The problem here, as with many other things, my focus was – and still is – on what I could do and what I can't do anymore. I should be grateful for being able to do the things I can do in the first place. I realise that when I am not trying to write, but when I am, it is a different story. The same thing happened with drawing. I loved drawing and used to do that very frequently, but like other things, that vanished as well. When I saw how hard writing was, I could not be bothered with drawing. Yes, this may seem a lazy and lousy excuse, but I would rather call it a psychological issue. I am a perfectionist; whenever I make a mistake or do something wrong, I freak out. It is not just when I am writing either, but in everything I do. If it were only a freak-out, everything would be fine, but I burst into tears, which later causes a headache.

Everything I could do, potentially can be described as lost. My parents, especially Dad, does not like that term. But I cannot see it any other way. If I walked around saying that I had gained things from my brain tumour, I would be fooling myself and others.

Another thing is that people would most definitely declare me as certifiable. I am aware of being negative here but let us be honest: if you are not able to do things you used to do, you have lost all those abilities, simple as that. No mystery there.

'Mostly it is loss which teaches us about the worth of things.'[16]

---

[16] Arthur Schopenhauer, German philosopher.

23

High School Loose Ends

◇

*The true measure of a man is how he treats someone who
can do him absolutely no good.*

~Samuel Johnson

In this chapter I explain everything about the matriculation
exam, which subjects were involved and why.

My high school report was not excellent so, in June 2003, three
months after my operation, I had to complete the matriculation test
at my school before I could graduate. I was fully aware of the fact
that it was all so fresh, and I was still recovering, but I felt totally fine
and not in any pain. The only issue was my independence – doing
things without the help of others. I cannot pinpoint the reason for
rushing and not waiting for the rehabilitation to end but knowing
myself, I just wanted to move my focus from recent happenings,
to shift my mind from the negativity, my possible death and the
aftermath I was left with. Doing so was beneficial for me in many

ways, mostly because I was replacing thoughts about what I'd been through with something enjoyable – learning.

The matriculation test consisted of two predetermined subjects and a subject of my choosing. The predetermined subjects were mathematics and Croatian language and literature. At the time, my Aunt Zvjezdana (Mum's cousin) was teaching three subjects at my school – ethics, sociology, and politics and economics. My mind was set on sociology. Apart from the fact my aunt could help me, I found it genuinely interesting. It is somewhat similar to psychology, which I found very interesting. I must note that I did not enrol in that school because of Aunt Zvjezdana. I did it because of my university plans and not to profit from my Aunt Zvjezdana as some people were suggesting. The best proof of this is that my school reports were not excellent throughout all four years. Of course, it was wonderful to have someone to turn to, but that is where it ended.

So, mathematics, Croatian language and literature, and sociology were my subjects for the matriculation test. I am kind of a nerdy person, so I do not like going to an exam unprepared. The embarrassment of not knowing is not my thing. I would rather spend the whole week glued to a book than to go through that uncomfortable situation. And above all, I am pretty attached towards being that nerdy persona, so losing my status was not an option. I love being that know-it-all person, so, I studied like crazy to pass the matriculation test and continue to university.

I was aware of the fact my surgery was just three months before the test. All my teachers were worried because it was so soon. But thankfully I could study, because I wanted to live up to my nerd reputation. First off was sociology. That was not hard, and it was interesting to me. It was an oral test that finished before it had even begun. I passed with no issues. Next was Croatian language and literature. Croatian language is easy when it comes to writing, because everything is written phonetically, the way it is pronounced. The problem is that the grammar rules are kind of chaotic. Not all, but some. I think it is in the first grade that pupils learn the additional letters in the Croatian alphabet. As I noted before, upon returning to Croatia, I enrolled in the second grade, because the Croatian and Australian education systems differ. Anyway, I missed out on learning the difference between *č* and *ć*, and when to use *ije* and *je*. They do not make sense to me, and I cannot seem to wrap my head around them. Luckily, there was not a lot of grammar on the test, so I passed it, no problem. The only bump, so to speak, was that my teacher that 'had to' diminish my grade. She was the class teacher who had visited me in the hospital. Out of all my teachers, she should have understood my situation. The reason for lowering my grade was literature. I had not read the book *Kiklop* by Ranko Marinković. I find her reason unimportant, especially because the rest of the class read that book while I had surgery, and I had been an A-grade student for all four years in her subject. *What's the big deal?*

The test saved the best for last – mathematics. I was terrified of my teacher. He was so strict. We classmates would joke that when we had his lesson, a person could hear a fly breathe. It was tombstone quiet! On the other hand, he was a magician. He had the ability to explain maths using daily experiences. I do not know how he managed to explain mathematical functions or logarithms using real-life examples. He explained maths in layman's term so that everyone could understand perfectly. I am talking about complicated maths, like functions, intervals and logarithms. A lot of students left school with a much better understanding of such subjects, thanks to him. Even though I was intimidated by him, looking back I can say that he was the best teacher I had throughout my whole education – primary school, secondary school, high school and university.

Getting back to the story, the maths exam was a written test, and I did not answer all the questions, so I was worried. I will never forget his words on the scoring: 'Colleague, I've been teaching you for four years now. I know exactly where you stand knowledgewise!' I was sitting in front of a real human being! A man who not only showed compassion and understanding but surpassed the meaning of this test and graded me by the knowledge I have shown during all four years of high school. I passed maths too. My overall score was excellent. The matriculation test was complete. That was done and dusted! Now I could concentrate on which university to choose in the given circumstances.

'Obstacles cannot stop you. Problems cannot stop you. Most of all, other people cannot stop you. Only you can stop you.'[17]

---

[17] Jeffrey Gitomer, American author, professional speaker and business trainer.

24

Appropriate University

◇

Adaptability is being able to adjust to any given situation at any given time.

~John Wooden

Finally, by March 2004, I had been free of cancer for a year, passed high school and was able to look after myself again. Everything was done according to my abilities, slowly and not in the same way that I used to do things, but independently. I reduced the number of remedies I used, but I still took vitamins and stuck to the Budwig diet. During that whole year – 2003 to 2004 – I think I overused everything – vitamins, different remedies and had had enough. I still exercised and walked, but I wanted to completely leave all the bad, the illness, behind me and go forward towards a new life. It was time to look to the future and choose a university.

My neurologist had to determine whether I could endure university in the first place. They had done some tests and it turned out that it would be very good for my brain to be occupied with study. But in consideration of what I'd had, I needed a calm and peaceful university, which meant nothing too demanding or stressful, without too many lectures per day. All my prior wishes and aspirations were abruptly expunged.

My initial wishes before all this happened had been to go to the University of Mechanical Engineering to study aviation, or to the University of Architecture. In the Faculty of Aviation, my speciality would be aircraft design. I really enjoyed technical drawing, so whichever of those two universities I got into was totally fine. The love for technical drawing ran in my blood; both Mum and her father were civil engineers.

That wish could not come to life because the tumour had left me with trembling and involuntary movements in my right hand. As my writing got better, I could draw but not as precisely or neatly as before. Being a perfectionist, it was very frustrating. I would often end up in tears. Given the fact that the tumour had already damaged my brain and body, to pursue technical drawing would be dangerous. I was to avoid stress and frustration, not add more and jeopardise my health.

I still wanted to study something. The urge to do so was overwhelming. At that time, I wanted to move on, forget. University was a way out for me, and if I add to that my thirst for knowledge, a perfect cocktail was concocted. Maybe psychology was a good option. I have always been interested in how the mind works and what determines our behaviour. I am aware that it is completely different from what I initially wanted to study, but nothing else clicked with me. Coincidentally, when the decision process was ongoing, I had an appointment with my neurologist. We spoke about psychology and my neurologist said that he would not recommend it. He said that it was not because of the difficulty, but because I needed to rest and take it slow. Psychology is too stressful, demanding, and my brain needed something light and easygoing. More rest, less effort.

After that meeting I was lost. All my aspirations had been dashed. I wanted to go to university, but it was very hard to find the one that ticked all the boxes I needed – well, the ones my wounded brain and body needed.

My parents and I looked at some brochures and saw some remarkably interesting combinations. One university offered a course where you choose from four subjects and combine two of them with each other or choose one and combine it to a detached course. The subjects were Croatian language and literature, history, philosophy, and teaching. The detached courses were Croatian language and literature, English language and literature, German language and literature and Information Science. In choosing subjects, I had three things in mind. First was the fact that I wanted to go to university. Second, I needed something to raise my spirits and distract me from the cancer cycle I was in. Third, that my aspirations were all cut, so I needed to choose the next best thing out of what was on offer.

Even though I'd been planning to go to either the University of Mechanical Engineering or University of Architecture since the eighth year of my schooling, I knew that the humanities suited me better than the sciences. This was reflected in my grades throughout primary, secondary and high school. My grades in humanities subjects such as history, geography, ethics and sociology were excellent, while science subjects such as mathematics, physics and chemistry were not so good.

In the university brochures, all the listed subjects were social sciences. That was a good thing because I knew I would be stressed out over grades. Also, all the subjects were easygoing and casual

– exactly what my brain and body needed. Apart from that, I had certain sympathies towards philosophy and thought that maybe history would be the most compatible of all with philosophy.

So, the decision was made. I would go to the University of J.J. Strossmayer in Osijek to study history and philosophy. Lectures began in September 2004. The university was not too far from my house, just five tram stops, so I would often walk home.

Looking back, I have no regrets about that decision because I found myself in those two subjects. Another plus was that I had an outlet for my drive to study and thirst for success. Apart from that, university proved to be beneficial for me in so many ways.

25

University Memories

◇

The roots of education are bitter,
but the fruit is sweet.

~Aristotle

I can clearly remember the first day of university. My feelings were a mix of anticipation, excitement and fear. Mostly fear. Fear that I would be a freak show waiting to happen. Fear that everyone would mock me because I came with my mother – she would write everything down and I would just sign. Fear that all of this would be too much for me…

My university acceptance letter had told me to arrive at the university's Grand Hall for eight a.m. on my first day. The hall was the size of a theatre and filled with hundreds of other nervous eighteen-year-olds. Truth be told, I was already twenty.

When all the students were seated, some documents had to be filled out, a process to get yourself established on their system. After that, the professor and his assistants gave us details about our courses: the times of classes, which group would attend which classes and when. They explained the rules regarding the signatures needed to access exams and all the other administration.

Although I was nervous, I was quite content and happy to be taking a new step in my life, a step away from my path of suffering and pain. I could shift my focus and occupy my mind with something other than tumours and death. I would gain knowledge and I love knowledge! Shifting your focus makes all the difference. I am saying that from the bottom of my heart. I have tested it. I know it. But the catch here is you must be interested. If you do it just because you want to avoid something bothering you or just for fun, you will fail. You need something strong enough to occupy you, to get glued to something, to make you give that something your full attention. That can only be attained through interest.

As days passed by, everyone showed that they were more interested in themselves and their own business. It was the opposite of high school, where everyone liked to know everyone else's business and teens can be so cruel. People grow up so much through primary school and high school that they do not need to mock or bully others. Well, that's true for most people. I was worried about those who had not grown up. Now, I can claim that my fears were completely unfounded, although I do know many people who are childish and do not act according to their age. Mistakes are a part of being human. Appreciate your mistakes for what they are – precious life lessons that can only be learnt the hard way.

Throughout my university years, I slowly became self-sufficient and independent to the point that I did not need help in any situation. I am very satisfied and grateful that I went to university. Not only did it give me knowledge, it also stopped me from feeling sorry about myself, from feeling unworthy, from feeling like a disabled person who needs pity. I was so consumed by studying and my other obligations that any negative feelings or fears vanished into thin air. Being a perfectionist who wants everything to be tip-top kept me away from dark thoughts. I did not even think about going into an exam without knowing at least ninety per cent of the theory. Mum always persuaded me to take an exam, you never know. But I would not budge. My thoughts about taking exams were that I do not like feeling uncomfortable and embarrass myself. Why would I want to disgrace myself? I understand that one cannot know everything but knowing more than average is my thing. Aim for the stars or in close proximity!

In saying that, I must retell a very awkward and lucky story. I was preparing for a particularly important exam on the history of the seventeenth and eighteenth centuries. Actually, I was more freaking out than preparing. It was an awfully hard exam, and, above all, it was mandatory to pass the year. In retrospect, a lot of the information given was unnecessary. The professors closely monitored how many students attended each lecture. Attendance was necessary in order to get the professor's signature so you could take the exam. They often used non-attendance to fail students. The final lecture of this subject was on an awful day. It was raining and cold outside, and I really did not want to go to it. But the more I thought about dropping out, the more some weird voice in my head was telling me to go. So, I went, and it turned out to be a lecture about Maria Theresa's fetish. The eighteenth-century queen of Hungary and Croatia was obsessed with underwear, especially panties. This information was not in our textbooks, so it turned out to be an essential lecture. This question would definitely be in the exam. Usually the lecture is an hour and a half, but this one was two hours and all about panties – colours, styles, the money she spent on them, her favourites... It was a little less dull than our usual seventeenth- and eighteenth-century history lectures although I am not completely sure what Maria Theresa's panties have to do with history! Maybe red panties meant war and white meant peace.

Anyway, the day of the exam came, and I was a complete mess, worrying that I did not know enough. The professor will surely dig up a question I do not know. As I walked into the professor's office, my mind calmed down. The exam was verbal, and my question was, 'Did Maria Theresa have any fetishes?' That was my only question, and I passed the exam with flying colours. Out of everything I learnt about the history of the seventeenth and eighteenth centuries, I remember panties the most.

The reason for mentioning this story is that it was a meaningful event for me. It showed me how things in life do not always happen as planned and sometimes you can get what you want with less or no effort involved. It was an eye opener!

My happiness and good fortune did not last long. As old people in my country say, tranquillity before the eruption. Misery was waiting just around the corner. If only happiness was so nice as to wait for you around the corner instead, or better yet, stayed with you.

26

The Recurrence

◇

Fortune knocks but once, but misfortune has much more patience.

~Lawrence J. Peter

*M*y university days flew by and before I knew it, the fourth year knocked on the door. Being a student meant so much to me on so many levels. Most of all, it distracted me from my old path and way of thinking. I was so consumed with studying and doing things related to university that all my worries and sorrows were washed away. It is amazing how doing something you are dedicated to turns your whole world around. My only goals were finishing my assignments and tying up all the loose ends regarding university.

Given the fact that my walking had improved, I did less and less formal exercise, just long walks. Sometimes I would walk home from university, but usually I used the tram, which still involved quite a bit of walking. The walking was beneficial for me; it was some form of workout after being cramped in a seat ninety minutes in lectures or seminars. But all in all, university was a huge plus for me, mentally, psychologically and physically.

May 2009 was nearing, which meant that my MRI test was coming up. But that did not worry me. My exams came first; everything else was less of a priority. The scan was scheduled for 5 May, and it had become routine for me. I did not like the routine, but it had to be done to be sure there were no malignant guests holidaying in my head or elsewhere.

On that day, I arrived at eight a.m., and the scan started. This time the scan was longer because they had to do my spine too. As I waited in the doctor's office to hear the results, I noticed the doctor was arguing on the phone with someone, visibly shaken. But it was of no concern to me. I just wanted to know the findings. Thankfully, the MRI was normal; my head and spine were clear. There were no signs of a relapse. Just as I expected! I was quite confident that the result would be fine, but still, that microgram of worry persisted.

After I was reassured that everything was fine, my studies continued freely. Near the end of my fourth year, one symptom occurred. My walking was a bit off. My usual walking gait was a bit faster because of momentum, but this was something else. I was tripping and sometimes it was quite difficult to keep myself from falling. I reminded myself that after the first operation my walking varied from excellent one day to bad the next. Plus, the MRI had been clear, so no worries. I figured that it was just a bad day and it would get better. My walking has been strange before. Why worry?

But as time passed, my walking worsened to the point where I could hardly stand. Soon after that, I started talking very slowly and had difficulty pronouncing certain words. It was obvious something was wrong. I needed to go to the hospital to sort things out. I saw millions of red neon lights and the word *RELAPSE* flashing on and off.

My mum tried to calm me. 'It's not a relapse, don't worry. The MRI was done days ago. Everything will be fine. Stressing will not help. Keep calm! I do not think it is a big deal. Because you are talking slowly and slurring your words, maybe it is just a mild stroke. We'll see!'

We went to the emergency neurological clinic because it was quicker than waiting for an appointment with my doctor. To my surprise, we came across a genuinely nice doctor, the total opposite of his colleagues. He was very attentive and understanding, but above all he knew his job. He examined me but said that it would be best to organise another MRI, so that we could rule out any head issues. We decided to find my radiologist while we were already at the hospital and schedule another MRI scan. The radiologist was reluctant at first. She said that it was quite normal to walk weirdly, given that there was a huge hole in my head from the first tumour and the immense summer temperatures outside.

Then Mum told her what she thought. 'Doctor, with all due respect, she was going to university with that hole and everything was fine. We've had hot days before and her walking was okay.'

After the persuasion, the radiologist finally agreed. 'Come early tomorrow. I'm on call, so I will squeeze you in.'

My psychological state was bad, a mixture of fear, frustration, anguish, and torment. Again, I fell into that dark hole of despair. Even university could not overcome this. When I commenced university, apart from the direction the university turned me to, I have to say that the 'must-do' MRI scans were not scary, dreadful or even hard to do. But in that moment of uncertainty all that changed. My mind was consumed by countless thoughts, all related to cancer. I could not quiet it, because I knew from my symptoms that something was going on. And as usual, the thoughts and emotions were not leaning towards positive outcomes. All of them were negative with no hope. I must admit that even in the moment I am writing these words, my stance is the same! Whenever something happens my mind always runs to dark, negative thoughts, and it is never a mild or modest negative thought. It is always the worst-case scenario. I do realise that the events of the past affected me, but it is not normal to think that a simple pain in a joint is bone cancer.

The new MRI was set for 28 May 2009. At least the scan was quick. In thirty minutes it was all finished. Then, we waited in pure agony for the results. After fifteen minutes, my mum could not wait any longer and decided to find the doctor. When she found her, the doctor told Mum that there was a small tumour, less than a centimetre in diameter. My second tumour was in the thalamus – a large mass of grey matter that relays sensory and motor signals to the cerebral cortex. It regulates consciousness, sleep, and alertness, and it was causing my current crop of symptoms.

Although it was only a few millimetres wide, it was still visible on the MRI I had had recently. I do not know why they had missed it. This oversight could have been fatal. My thoughts about doctors are well known, but still! If I did not have that experience of horrible doctors' charades prior, it would almost be funny. How on earth is it possible that doctors in the twenty-first century, with sophisticated and advanced devices, can miss a tumour? Even now, I sometimes cannot believe it.

27

Preliminary Meeting

◇

*Sometimes the best thing you can do is not think, not
wonder, not imagine and not obsess. Just breathe and
have faith that everything will work out for the best.*

~Unknown

*O*n hearing the news that my cancer was back, we decided
to go to my neurologist to ask for guidance. I sat in the
hospital hallway while my mum went to find her. After a couple
minutes, Mum came back, visibly shaken. She said the doctor's
exact words were, 'Okay, it's a relapse. So what are you doing here?
Go where you resolved the first one!' Where are medical ethics?
Where is the Hippocratic Oath? Where is her humanity? The doctor's response was devastating.

During this time, my dad was in Australia working as a carpenter in different venues. Carrying a phone to work was prohibited for safety reasons. He returned from work that day to a flurry

of messages and missed calls. He immediately realised something was wrong. When he received the news, he packed up his things and scheduled a flight for Croatia.

In the meantime, Mum and I were struggling. This recurrence shattered us. All the precautions I had taken and made had been in vain. We could not find a light. Any kind of positivity was far, far away. After some time, we managed to compose ourselves. It was not the time for despair, heartbreak or negativity; some serious action was needed. Only then would it be possible for me to overcome this. We decided to get in contact with Dr Angel. Mum called Rebro in Zagreb and reached his secretary. She told us she could not organise an appointment because Dr Angel was too busy.

The secretary said, 'Maybe if you called him directly, you would have more luck.' So, Mum called the man who put us in touch with Dr Angel the first time. He managed to organise a meeting for us. *That man is truly awesome!*

In the meantime, my dad arrived back in Croatia. This homecoming was not joyful at all, unlike his previous ones, but when he saw us at Zagreb airport, he was relieved. I think the fact that we were together calmed him. We returned to our house in Osijek and filled him in on the situation.

We sadly reunited with Dr Angel on 20 June 2009. He told us that the new tumour was in a very awkward place in the brain called the thalamus, a small structure located just above the brain stem, between the cerebral cortex and the midbrain. Operating on the thalamus would be, in his words, 'Like letting an elephant walk into a glass room. It is an extremely sensitive area in the brain permeated with nerves. If the nerves are touched, the consequences would be enormous!'

'There is another approach', he continued, 'Gamma Knife surgery.[18] It is a relatively new technique in Croatia, about four years old. Only a few hospitals have this type of surgery. It is a kind of radiosurgery where intense cobalt radiation is administered over a small area. I believe that this radiosurgery is the best in this case and most efficient. It is designed for tumours smaller than four centimetres, and this one is less than one centimetre big. A friend of mine, Dr Saviour, is practising it. He is more than satisfied with the results. It has been proven to help with and destroy brain tumours that are otherwise hard to reach or are inoperable.'

After hearing this, I felt a tiny bit better. At least there would be no classic operation. As satisfied as I was, different questions started to pile up. Crucially, would the new method be as efficient and helpful as traditional surgery? I had heard everything he had said and it all made sense, but still that worm of doubt did not go away. It is not that I did not trust my doctor. It is just a primitive fear all humans have regarding something new. Sticking to the old and well-established way feels better than welcoming in the new. It is ironic: I do not think like that when it comes to technical innovations that make life easier. I guess the line is drawn when it comes to living or dying.

Dr Angel somehow detected this and started reassuring me. 'This is a much better procedure and much safer. There is no invasion of the brain like there is in classic surgery. Cobalt beams do all the work, so no opening of the skull is required. Plus, I do not think you have any other option. It is either this or a classic

---

[18] The Gamma Knife, also known as the Leksell Gamma Knife, is a type of radiation surgery. It is used to treat brain tumours by administering high-intensity cobalt radiation in a concentrated dose over a small area. It aims to deliver an ablative dose of radiation in a single treatment session, while sparing surrounding tissues.

operation, and we are certain of the outcome there. Of course, if you refuse both procedures, there is the option of alternative medicine. But if you agree to this radiosurgery, I will call Dr Saviour to schedule a meeting for you.'

In the end, I agreed. What choice did I have? The fact that I could end up stuck in a bed for the rest of my life from classic surgery terrified me. This procedure did not guarantee a good outcome or smooth recovery, but it was worth a try.

As it turned out, Dr Saviour was free, so we could meet him immediately. He too, assured us that Gamma Knife surgery was the best way to go. Best of all, he told me that I would not have to stay in hospital at all.

'The procedure is done in a day. You do not have to stay in the hospital. When everything is finished you can go home. The radiation treatment is delivered with great precision to the target tissue within the brain, while at the same time minimising any dose to surrounding healthy tissue.'

Of course, there was a downside. Dr Saviour went on to discuss the aftermath. 'After the procedure, a patient usually gets an oedema due to the intensity of the radioactive cobalt beamed into the brain. Oedema is a sort of reaction from the brain.[19] To resolve this, corticosteroid injections are given to reduce the inflammation. The dose starts high and will be tapered off slowly. We will calculate the exact dose and get back to you. It all depends on the oedema and how big it is. These injections can be given to Tihana

---

[19] Cerebral oedema is swelling caused by a build-up of fluid in the spaces of the brain. This typically causes impaired nerve function, increased pressure within the skull and can eventually lead to direct compression of brain tissue and blood vessels. It can be fatal.

by her GP. The radiosurgery does not take effect immediately. You will feel the effects of it in about three months."

The surgery was scheduled for 26 June 2009. This time there was no preparation. I just needed to show up. There were no pre-operative procedures to do, so that made everything easier. My only 'chore' was surviving the days to the procedure.

I was content that it was not a classic, open-brain surgery, but I was full of fear and negative thoughts about the final outcome. Yes, Dr Angel did calm me regarding the radiosurgery and Dr Saviour's words reassured me, but I was still worried. This was not normal worry; this was panic worry. I understood this was a better and safer way to kill the tumour. But nonetheless, I was terrified. I could not believe the cancer could be destroyed by lying down for thirty minutes. I was aware that a large amount of radiation was used to kill it, but I could not wrap my head around it. The procedure seemed too good to be true. Along with that, I was also worried about what would happen over the next three months. Putting it plainly, how is it possible that for the first three months after the procedure I would be able to walk and everything would be okay, then, after three months, I wouldn't be able to walk and everything would be altered? It does not make sense!

University and all the effort I had put into it went down the drain. AGAIN!!! My aspirations towards a new future after surviving the first operation were destroyed with no return. Overcoming the initial tumour and its aftermath had been exceedingly difficult and draining. But after that, I commenced university and slowly started sorting out my thoughts, diet, and behaviour ready for a new future that did not include cancer or any other health issues. The support and compassion I received for this first tumour was great and really helped. But the consolation I felt was limited. After all, I was the one who must deal with radiosurgery and with whatever the cancer left behind. It was a horrible, terrifying period of six days that I do not like remembering.

My parents' overall state did not differ much from mine. The only difference was that they firmly believed in the radiosurgery Dr Saviour would perform. This was because they both trusted Dr Angel's methods. He would not advise us to do radiosurgery were it not the best option. They were both inconsolable, but neither Mum nor Dad feared for one moment that I would die.

28

Gamma Knife

◇

We may stumble and fall but shall rise again; it should be
enough if we did not run away from the battle.

~Mahatma Gandhi

We decided to go to Zagreb for the Gamma Knife surgery a day early to be well rested and ready, so there would be no rush and stress. It was a four-hour drive from Osijek to Zagreb, and the procedure was scheduled for eight a.m. Apart from wanting to avoid worry and stress, several other things needed to be done, like managing the food for the day, and after that, finding a motel or hotel near Rebro Hospital and finalising all the paperwork.

We arrived at the Gamma Knife ward an hour before the procedure was due to start. A nurse came to us and said that I should start the preparation. Preparation? What in the world could she mean by that? Remembering the anaesthesia debacle, I instantly thought maybe they wanted to insert different fluorescent tubes in my brain to make the procedure more fun to look at. I am joking but judging from my experience with anaesthesia last time, I do not think I am too far off. Fearing what to expect, I followed her like a child going to get a flu shot. The nurse and I entered a room where an awkward-looking mask sat on the table. The table was in the centre of the room, surrounded with different shelves, draws and cupboards. At first, I had the feeling I was in a museum viewing archaeological findings The reason for this was a mask which was illuminated on the table. For a moment, I remembered the movie *The Man in the Iron Mask* and remembered how I kind of had a crush on Leonardo DiCaprio.

The nurse brutally cut off my daydream and explained, 'It's not a mask because it doesn't cover the face. You could call it a kind of helmet. It directs the cobalt beams into the tumour precisely. We have to position it correctly. To check that, we will use the MRI.' *As if I cannot get enough of that dreadful machine.*

Another nurse came, and together, they positioned the helmet on my head and then affixed it with five or six flat-ended screws. At first it did not hurt, but as the screws came closer to my scalp – oh dear! Not only did it hurt, it felt as though they were drilling the screws into my head. Awful! When the helmet was screwed on, they sent me for an MRI. I had never had a scan in the Rebro Hospital before because all my earlier scans were done at the hospital in Osijek. They gave me earplugs for the scan because the MRI was extremely loud. Apart from dealing with the stillness, an added feature was the noise. The earplugs were not effective. I still felt as though I was on a plane runway.

The scan showed that the position of the helmet was off by a fraction of a millimetre, so they had to re-adjust it. The second time was successful. These preparations took a couple of hours.

Immediately, the image of the anaesthesia fiasco came vividly to mind again as we ran back and forth adjusting the helmet.

Finally, the Gamma Knife surgery began. It is remarkably similar to an MRI, only the machine is shorter and quieter. The patient lies down as if for an MRI but this time only the head and upper chest are in the tube, as opposed to an MRI where the whole body is in the tube. The whole procedure lasted for about an hour and twenty minutes. Again, like the MRI, I needed to keep as still as possible while the machine did its job. At least I am used to that, but my head was in overdrive with all different thoughts. *Will the tumour be destroyed? How will the procedure be done? Will it be efficient?* In that moment, in the machine with my helmet on, I ordered myself to stop thinking, to change my focus.

Then a thought, both funny and sad, came up. My peers brag about their familiarity with driving, sex and other hedonistic pleasures, while here I am bragging about being familiar with MRI scans. *Rotten luck!*

The whole radiosurgery procedure was over in about two or three hours. All in all, the surgery did not take long. The preparations – putting on the mask and checking whether it was adjusted correctly – took most of the time. The actual Gamma Knife took thirty to thirty-five minutes.

When the procedure was over, we went to see the Dr Saviour. It had been successful as far as his team could tell at this point, but we needed to wait and see. Dr Saviour told us, 'An MRI will show how successful the procedure was. Schedule one in three months' time. You do not need to come here. You can do it in Osijek and email the results to me.'

I hoped the results would be known sooner. At least after the first surgery, I immediately knew whether it had been successful or not. This time, I had to wait and hope for a good outcome. I might be a little naughty, but after the first tumour, I got used to the fact that the results were available immediately. As I was well known in the Osijek Hospital, my radiologist was kind enough to let me in on the results before they were printed out.

Then Dr Saviour continued, 'Tihana will develop cerebral oedema, a brain swelling. She will need corticosteroid injections to reduce the swelling. These injections can be given to Tihana by her GP.'

I did not want to interrupt him, but I could not wait anymore. I quickly jumped in and asked if the procedure had worked or not, because nothing had changed. My body felt the same.

He replied, 'No, it's currently not working. You will see its effects in three months or so. It will be gradual. You will have to be calm and composed. Arm yourself with patience!'

Then, my Mum asked about the recovery process.

He said, 'I'm not going to lie to you. We do not actually know how the body will react and what the consequences will be. But I am certain strong will and endurance are your best and only options. If you combine those two with physiotherapy, you have three enormously powerful instruments. Focus on them, and you can create wonders.'

His words gave me unusual power and determination to fight and conquer my situation. Even now writing this, I must admit that my battle was and still is long, fatiguing, frustrating, dull. Sometimes I feel there is no use trying or fighting or hoping. Let me just lie down and die. But then it occurs to me that awaiting death would be an even more nerve-racking process. I have no option other than to fight my battle and hope for the best outcome. At that point, I did not have a clue what to expect – mild, medium, or severe changes in my abilities. But one thing was crystal clear: I could not run away from myself or the situation I was in.

When life gets hard, you can quit or go on with the battle. In doing so, one must weigh the pros and cons of both options. I am saying this because in my situation I was confronted with a lot of pros in quitting and a lot of cons in continuing the battle.

29

The Oedema Fiasco

◇

Be sure you put your feet in the right place,
then stand firm.

~Abraham Lincoln

fter the radiosurgery procedure was done, we headed straight home. When we got there, my overall state – physical and psychological – seemed to be picture perfect. At least that was what my movements and everything else indicated. My speech, my writing, my hand movements and my walking were the same as after the first operation. Not even one part of my body was showing any changes.

Regarding remedies and vitamins, of all the different remedies I had tried after my first operation, only the Budwig diet was still in use. Frankly, this remedy sits so well with me that I do not think I will stop it any time soon. I increased the number of vitamins I was already taking. The gist of it all is that I continued with vitamin usage as well as the Budwig diet. I really do believe in the power of vitamins. Of course, they do not take immediate effect but in the long term they work wonders.

My hometown of Osijek is inland, so my parents and I decided to go to Dalmatia for a nice holiday. It was the end of June and beginning of July, so summer in Croatia. Usually every year or two, we would go there for a holiday. We did not have a routine place to go. We would see where we ended up. Dalmatia is a coastal part of Croatia, and tourism is highly developed. Most people who live there depend on the income from tourism.

Anyway, during our holiday, I noticed mild walking problems starting to re-surface. Some steps were okay, but some were a challenge. Also, I would lose my balance. At first it was rare but as time moved on, it got more frequent. Short walks to the shop or the beach were not a problem. The issues appeared in the evenings when we would go for long walks on the seafront. The issues were not big but they cut the walks short. In time, I got used to the fact that my walking was not so good. Despite all of this, the holiday was very relaxing, exactly what all of us needed.

Apart from the enjoyment and rest I got from the holiday, as Dr Saviour promised, the radiosurgery started working while we were away. Upon coming back home to Osijek, I had an MRI scan that showed brain swelling, the cerebral oedema he had warned us about. I needed to start taking corticosteroids injections. Cerebral oedema, as noted previously, is when fluid builds up around the brain, causing an increase in intracranial pressure (ICP). ICP can affect the whole brain or specific regions depending on the underlying cause. Cerebral oedema can cause irreversible damage and, in some cases, be fatal. So, to avoid this I had to take appropriate measures – corticosteroids injections.

This straightforward health requirement caused all hell to break loose in the doctors' world in my hometown. It was a soap opera. 'Days of Our Lives' and 'The Bold and the Beautiful' were plain sitcoms compared to this. The corticosteroids needed to be injected by my GP three times a week, for three weeks. The dose started at fourteen millilitres and would gradually be reduced.

Once we had all this information from Dr Saviour, Mum contacted my GP. I think if she had contacted the devil himself, she would have had a better run. The GP, aka Dr Hell, was polite and helpful at first, but as time passed, her transformation astonished me.

The first issue was that I could not walk upstairs, and her office was on the first floor in a building without a lift. But, as she had an obligation to do house calls, we thought that everything would be fine. She could come to my house. She seemed okay with this arrangement. The emphasis here is on *seemed*; in reality, she was beyond furious. As time passed, her disapproval became more and more evident. Eventually, she refused to come to my house. She decided the car park in front of her practice was a suitable place for that non-invasive medical procedure – a pleasant situation with people passing and looking while Dr Hell gave me an injection in the bum. Unfortunately, even that started to present a problem for her. At that moment, I was totally lost for words. I did not know whether to laugh or cry. Now, looking back, I am saddened and demoralised by it. Where does vanity stop, and medicine begin for doctors? We were hoping she would at least finish giving me the injections, even if it was in the car park. But at the beginning of the second week of my regime, Mum received a rather disturbing phone call from the man, who ran another clinic in Osijek. We had never been to that clinic. He did not know me, Mum or Dad.

This man verbally bashed my Mum. 'Who do you think you are? How can you expect a GP to do home visits? A GP is not bound to do this! Your GP has other patients and is too busy to do home visits.'

My mother, visibly shaken, called Dr Saviour to ask what to do. She got in touch with his secretary who was also upset because the same man had had the nerve to call Dr Saviour in Rebro too. A short time after that, Dr Saviour got on the line. Mum started apologising for the unpleasant situation caused by that man and the trouble we were in.

Dr Saviour assured Mum that everything will be okay. 'Measures will be taken to resolve this situation. I am furious! He will be reported to the medical board for this. Doctors are obliged to do house visits. Do not worry. Everything will be sorted out.'

Shortly afterwards, my mum received another phone call. It was that man again. 'Hello, Mrs Babic. I am calling just to tell you everything is alright. Your daughter will continue getting the injections at home. We are sorry for the previous inconvenience. In the future, should there by anything your daughter might require, be sure to contact me.'

Later, we learnt the real reason of his first call. Through a family connection, we discovered he was in a romantic relationship with Dr Hell. He wanted to be perceived as her knight in shining armour, so he attacked my mum. Trying to prove his loyalty by being his lover's hero.

Sometimes I am still astonished by all of this. I still cannot believe that things like this happen.

30

Aftermath

Miracles come in moments.
Be ready and willing.

~Wayne Dyer

When we got home from Dalmatia in mid-September, the widespread effects of the Gamma Knife surgery started showing in every physical, and sometimes psychological, aspect of my being. I was back in my dear friend's arms again – the wheel-chair. This aftermath was very similar to what I had experienced following the first operation. I am certain that the intense radiation caused this change.

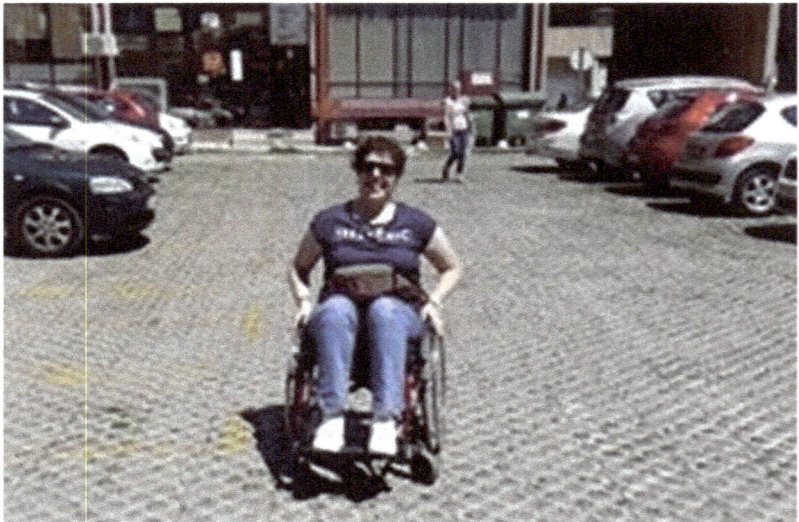

After the Gamma Knife

Some of the aftermath effects were mild and they would quickly pass, while others were awfully hard and painful. I suffered pins and needles throughout my whole left side. Even as I am writing this, I feel them. The intensity has declined but they are present. I have learnt to live with that feeling. In saying this, I have no idea if or when the pins and needles sensation is going to stop or whether I will feel them for the rest of my life. I experienced headaches in a periodic cycle. Vision wise, my eyesight was unchanged. I had worn glasses for near-sightedness since my first tumour. My hearing had not got any worse since the first tumour. It was still severely damaged on the right side. My vision and hearing issues had dragged on from the first tumour to the second one. At least they did not change! I have had problems with swallowing since the first operation. The recurrence only made things worse. After the second tumour, I developed extensive saliva leakage.

It feels like someone left the faucet on. Speech wise, it did not change too much for better or worse. My speech stayed the same – slow. Maybe it improved a little because I was not dragging words like I used to.

The sensations in my hands were not the same for the left and right. My right hand could easily distinguish different materials from one another. With my left hand, everything felt the same, nothing could be distinguished. The odd thing was, I could feel hot or cold but with that came erratic movements. When I touched something hot with my left hand it would draw back uncontrollably – hitting or knocking over anything in its path. It did not even have to be burning hot. My hand did the same with warm objects or semi-hot ones. My sense of touch had been altered. I was unable to write with my left hand. I am naturally right-handed but after the first operation, I learnt to write with my left hand because I developed a tremor in my right. This time round, the tremor in my right hand had reduced, only for the left to start shaking.

My ataxia – the loss of voluntary muscle coordination – once again arose after it had eventually disappeared following my first tumour. As I mentioned previously, I lost the ability to walk and found myself wheelchair-bound. I used to see the world from 178 centimetres; now it was down to 120 centimetres. *Bummer!*

At first, all of this was overwhelming. I was psychologically crushed. I realised I had been in this state before, yet I was inconsolable. I was tired and did not want to deal with all this. And the doctor's charade did not help. It only made everything more difficult. But I need to wake up and take some steps in regard to my situation. Okay, so I had some adapting to do. This set-up was familiar to me from my first brain tumour. The only difference would be the duration. Before, the set-up went away quickly. From what I could tell this time, from the reactions and movements of my body, this was not going away so soon. My limbs were stiff and hard to move, and my body felt weird. It was as if my head and legs were disconnected from my trunk, each with a mind of its own. I lost all coordination. I felt like a three-part alien. My head wanted to have coffee; my trunk wanted to chill; my arms wanted to do crafting; and my legs wanted to play tennis. Very weird. It was hard to unite them into one, and that created a big issue.

I am giving you a sneak peek into my life after the recurrence. There are times when I am so tired, my eyes do not cooperate. Double vision makes it hard to read. If I do not sleep enough, I get awfully bad headaches. It would be incredibly challenging to play a game where both hands were required as they have no synchronicity whatsoever. Do not even get me started on walking. The non-walking element has been present since 2009 and still persists.

The aftermath really sucks!

The question of physiotherapy arose. After the first operation, my rehabilitation was relatively quick, and I did not require help. Everything could be accomplished alone – feeding, dressing, washing, walking independently. The aftermath of the radiosurgery was different, more complex. Seeing my ataxia and lack of walking, we needed to act. We could tell from my movements that performing my exercises would not be enough. I had to seek help from a professional if I wanted good results. Since then, I have been battling to find the right physiotherapist.

It all started in 2009 with a rehabilitation centre called Lječilište Bizovačke Toplice, some fifteen to twenty kilometres from Osijek. The institution was like the rehabilitation centre in Krapina, but its focus on therapy differed. While the one in Krapina focused on post-surgery therapy, this one was more physiotherapy oriented. I started doing exercises there, but they were not the kind of exercises I needed.

We did some research online and found something called the Bobath Concept. The Bobath Concept is a neurological rehabilitation protocol, used in stroke patients and children with cerebral palsy. We found out my physiotherapist at Lječilište Bizovačke Toplice was a beginner in Bobath, so I stayed there six or so months hoping that maybe he'd get better. Later, he told us about a Bobath physiotherapist in Zagreb who was more knowledgeable about the different exercises and techniques. So, we started going there, to Reactiva in Zagreb. We went there every two months for sixteen or seventeen days at a time. While there, I had exercises daily, excluding weekends, for six hours, sometimes more. The hours included two hours with a specialised Bobath physiotherapist, two hours with a masseuse and two hours or more in the gym. This went on for a year and a half. It was hard but I endured it. That was my only option. I had to keep on for my own wellbeing.

Six or seven months after the radiosurgery and my MRI was due. I was physically and mentally wrecked, but curious about the results. It was done in the hospital in Osijek and happily only lasted thirty minutes because only my brain was scanned. The results were astonishing! The tumour was gone. It had totally vaporised. The Gamma Knife only kills the tumour by disabling the tumour cells; it does not remove the tumour. The dead tumour cells stay in the brain. Except, in my case there was just an empty space. The tumour had disappeared! No one knows how, or what happened. It is a medical phenomenon. Dr Saviour said that this was the first time something like this had happened. He had never come across anything similar working in Croatia and prior to that, the United States. Upon reading my scans, he immediately called Mum and asked if he could show them to the students he teaches. Mum told me and asked if I was willing to share my case. I joyfully agreed. What a beautiful miracle!

31

University Loose Ends

◇

Education is the most powerful weapon which you can use to change the world.

–Nelson Mandela

*T*ime was slowly but surely elapsing since the Gamma Knife surgery. My state was unchanged. Thankfully nothing deteriorated further than what I noted in the previous chapter. This was quite enough to deal with. I am not sure whether I could cope with more issues. Choking, saliva, headaches, being wheelchair-bound, ataxia. Dealing with that day in and day out. Adding to that, exercise. But this was not enough, so I have been given a bonus – psychological issues. Again thankfully, there were not as many, as there had been after the first operation. I was 'excluded' from depression and deep negativity as time went on.

At first, right after the Gamma Knife, I was depressed – in the state *why again? Will it stop?* But somehow, I managed to pull myself out of that dark hole, filled with despair, negativity and self-pity. I do not know how or what helped. It just happened. There still were days where all that negativity and misery would catch me. When that happened, I would be in deep – feeling sorry for myself, the persistent *why me* questions, sorrow, despair. All the negative emotions were present. Except suicide! I'm filled with gratitude for that! My stance regarding suicide is well known. It cannot be justified. It's an act of cowardice that I do not approve of. I think my belief served me in terms of not thinking about it. And I think that the loose end helped, in terms of changing my focus. Not finishing university affected me. Not in terms of anything bad, I just like finishing what I have started. I do not like unfinished business, never did!

Because of my relapse, my university education had abruptly stopped in its fourth year. I needed to complete one more year in order to graduate – the practical experience. The educational system in Croatia follows the Bologna Process[20], which seeks to bring coherence and standardisation to higher education systems across Europe. In participating countries, it takes three years to earn a bachelor's degree and five years for a master's. As I said, my study was cut short in the fourth year. I had one more year of practical experience left. This differs from subject to subject. In my case, studying history and philosophy, the praxis included a minor number of seminars, but mainly going to classrooms, listening to lectures or doing the lectures yourself. That is considered a test for which you get a certain grade. I was excluded from the praxis because of what happened. It was a good thing too, because it would have been a big struggle for me to attend classes in different schools in my situation. The practical experience covers visiting different schools and adapting to diverse classrooms. So, to get my MA, I just needed to pass my fourth year and write my thesis.

---

[20] The Bologna Process established the European Higher Education Area to facilitate student and staff mobility, and to make higher education more inclusive and accessible throughout Europe.

I chose to write about 9/11. Even though it had happened ten years earlier, I was still obsessed by it. The thought of a plane slamming into a building seemed astonishing to me. I wanted to study that topic. Even though there is a lot of controversy surrounding that topic, I needed to stick to the official report.

It was a good time to move my focus from my illness to a more positive path. University once again lifted me up. Being engaged in studying and research got me out of bed in the morning, even though my rehabilitation was ongoing.

The exams were so hard. Any hope I had that the professors would cut me some slack because of my situation was an illusion. They drilled me like any other student. To be quite honest, that was what I wanted. I did not want to be a Master of Education in History and Philosophy just for the title. I wanted to have some knowledge behind it. My wish was granted!

I graduated on 29 June 2011. Everyone was dressed in graduation gowns and caps. Even though I was in wheelchair, it was a wonderful and formal event. *So proud!*

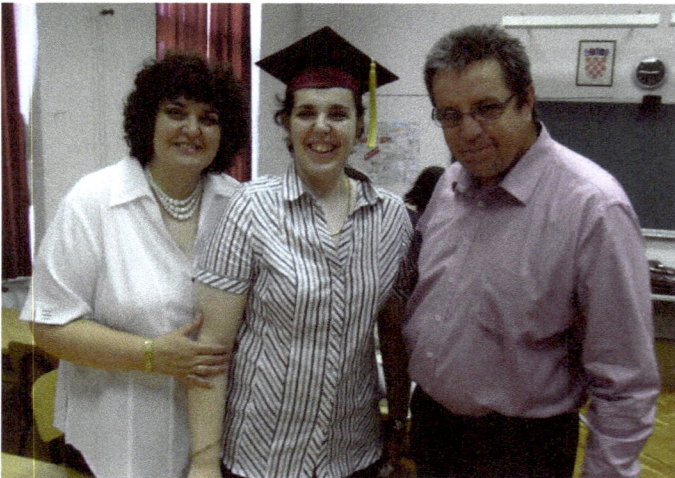

Master of History and Philosophy

32

The Land Down Under

◇

If you are brave enough to say goodbye, life will reward you with a new hello.

–Paulo Coelho

After university, things calmed down and I returned to my routine way of life that included exercise and relaxation. Exercise consisted of home training – things to keep me fit and moving. Relaxation was a bit of everything – sitting in my backyard and doing crosswords, TV, playing on my laptop, doing puzzles, building models. My schedule was only full-on when we went to Reactiva. Thanks to my Mum's cousin Sanda and her husband Damir, we had a place to stay for free in Zagreb. They are professors and they really understood me. My profession is a teacher also, even though I never worked, so my time in Zagreb combined business and pleasure.

As time went on, going to Australia, specifically to Western Australia (WA), was on our minds. Ever since we returned to Croatia in 1992, my dad had been commuting back and forth between Croatia and WA. In Croatia, he would mainly rest or do some carpentry work. In WA, he was a carpenter working in various places in north WA as a fly-in, fly-out worker.

Fly-in fly-out is a method of employing people in remote areas by flying them temporarily to the work site instead of relocating employees and their families permanently. It is often abbreviated to FIFO. It is common in large mining regions in Australia and Canada. It was a bit of a struggle for Mum and me on one side and Dad on the other. The separation and huge distances were hard to endure. At this point nothing was preventing Mum and me from joining Dad in WA. Of all the obstacles in our path, only Mum's job was left. My health issues were thankfully over. Everything was calming down. I only had the aftermath left to deal with. At that time, I was 'blessed' with fewer issues than today. But more of that later.

My dad had a very good friend, Frank, in WA. They were constantly talking about Mum and me coming to WA. He mentioned a house his parents owned. It had been renovated recently and was ready for new tenants.

When Dad returned home sometime around June 2013, we thoroughly discussed moving to WA. When I say 'we', I mean Mum and Dad, because I was physically present but, in some ways, I was not there. It is awkward to explain. I was like a child who does not have a say. My parents, of course, asked for my opinion. I answered that I agreed to go, but it was because I could not conceive of the idea of them not being by my side. It was like my body was twenty-nine years old, but my mind was only ten. I was not concerned about their service, them waiting on me: my worries were *what would I do without them? How would I survive?* I needed their comfort, their understanding, their presence in general. I felt like a minor who needs their parents. *Sometimes still do!*

When I was at my psychiatrist's establishing whether I was well enough for university, she told us about the possibility of the brain tumour affecting my emotions. She said that a brain tumour can influence the brain to the point that the patient is left at the emotional level of a child. After the first tumour, I did not have that feeling, but after the second tumour I experienced it. Along with the feeling of being 'asleep'. This feeling is particularly weird and hard to understand. I don't know what words to use to explain what I felt or how it affected me. In trying to make it comprehensible, I was oblivious to everything else except my misfortune and the aftermath. I think that the feeling lingered from 2009 to 2015. It was only then when I 'woke' from my slumber that I was aware and vigilant. A contradictory but absolutely true experience.

Anyway, Frank told Dad that he needed to contact his parents about the details of the rent. Once everything was settled and arranged, we started packing.

The more I thought about moving back to Australia, the better I felt about the idea. My stance was that WA would be a fresh page, a new start. I passionately believed that Australia would be a cancer-free country for me. No more illness. No more health struggles from the time we landed in Australia onwards.

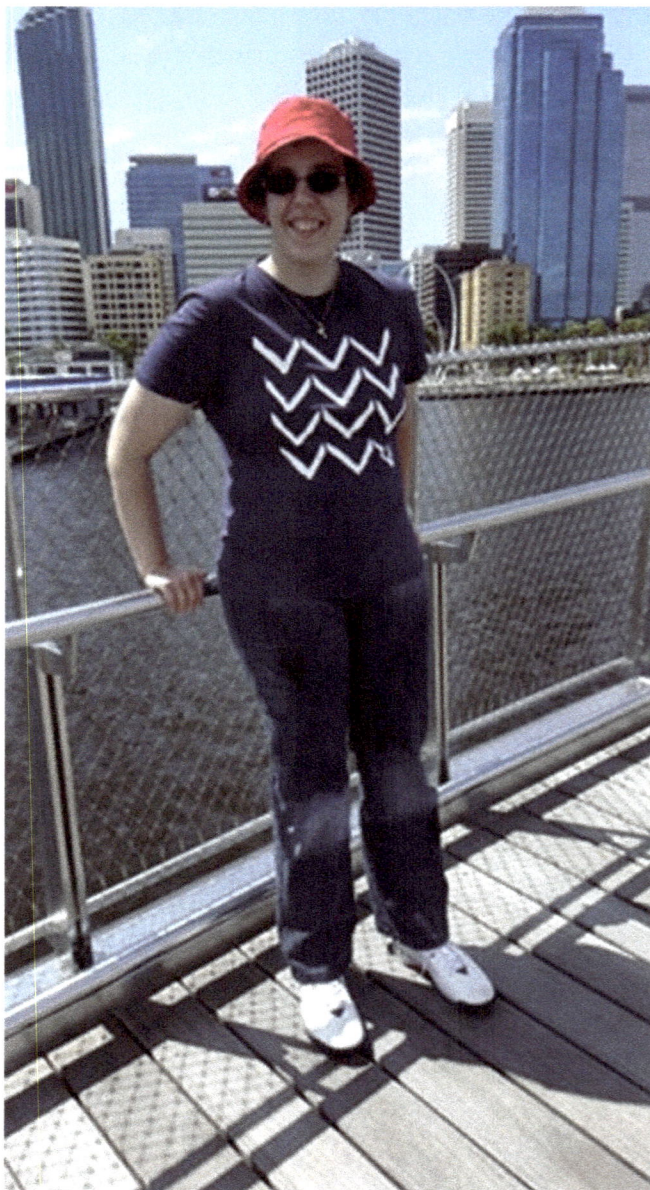

Perth, Western Australia – Chilling in the sun

A year has passed in WA, and a new chapter in my life is unfolding. I must admit that moving here was beneficial in so many ways, primarily, getting me out of the dark hole I was in. Do not misunderstand, I still have my moments of frustration, anger, rage, asking 'why did this happened to me?' or similar questions. It is a lot better now than in Croatia where it was more frequent and evident. But my main problem remains – not overcoming what happened, not accepting and not taking responsibility for it. This burden or history from my point of view is so vivid and so present that I feel as if it cannot be erased or diminished in my mind. I guess my only friend in that area is time. Whining and pining about my situation will not help. It will only make things worse.

On a more pleasant note, I think that Australia is slowly healing my wounds. The time spent here and the easygoing way of life in this country is making me forget and move forward to the future. I developed a much happier and positive way of thinking. That shift of focus and viewing things differently came from the extreme generosity and helping hand Australia gave me. The care, help, nourishment is enormous – out of this world! From the moment I arrived in Australia, I was taken care of and considered as if I had never left in the first place. Being a citizen is one thing, but receiving all this after twenty-one years of being away speaks volumes about this country. Immense gratitude!

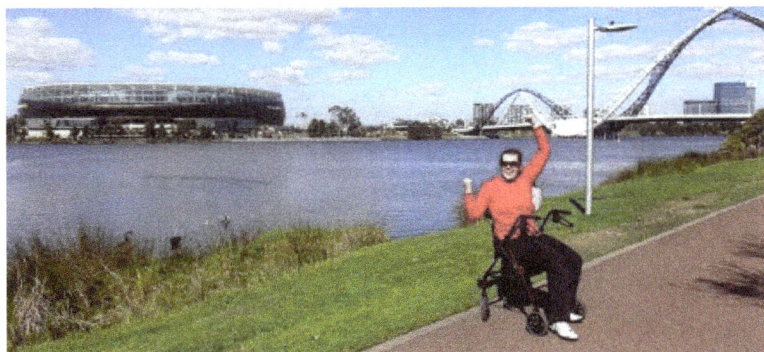

East Perth adventures

In those early days, the question of disability support arose. Wheelchair-bound, with all those side effects, I could not work or look for a job so we started applying for the disability pension. Initially, receiving the pension payment was impossible because of our residency status in Australia. But luckily, the Australian government agreed to accept that period we lived in Australia before, from May 1988 to November 1992. Sadly, even that was not enough: ten years of residency was required. The Australian government agency dealing with my case did not want to leave me without financial help, so they put me on the Newstart allowance until I would be eligible for the disability pension. I needed to report every fortnight to let them know I hadn't done any work. That lasted until July 2019 when I was permitted to get the disability pension. Now I am excluded from reporting and keep in mind that I must contact them for any changes in my life.

As we spent time in Australia, it became quite clear we would not go back to Croatia. There were several reasons for that, including the family impact the distance caused and the fact that we had sold our house in Croatia. We decided to start house hunting. Given the fact that we resided in Hamilton Hill in Western Australia and had adapted to the area, we began our search in that region. First off, the idea of buying an already built house persisted. Mum and Dad thought that they would adapt the house to our requirements and that would be it. We visited so many houses, but none suited us. Then we realised that an old house will always be an old house no matter how much you renovate it, and when an old house is bought, additional money will need to be spent down the line to restore it. Therefore, building a new house was our new goal. After seeing different potential land blocks, we – as a family – finally approved of one land block that was only five streets from the house we were renting. Within a year, our new house was built by one of the construction companies in WA.

When we settled in our new house, I started looking for physiotherapist. Very shortly, I began working with a physiotherapist named Zhao. He's a miracle worker. That man taught me so many things but above all he knew his job extremely well. We have worked together for five years and I deeply cherish the things I have learnt from him. This may seem like bragging, but truthfully, I have never come across a physiotherapist quite like him, and I have worked with countless. He is an exceptionally good physiotherapist and person!

33

Gamma Knife Legacy

◇

The river is wild. You cannot control it.
Embrace the chaos.

~Maxime Lagacé

After two years of life in Australia, the Gamma Knife showed its ugly face once again. As I noted before, from the moment the radiosurgery started working, I felt pins and needles in my left side, more in my left hand and left foot than anywhere else. My life continued despite that – exercising, training, trying to walk. And then around May 2015, something started happening. My ability to speak slowly began deteriorating. I did not know why but I started poking my tongue out when I was talking and that was making it difficult for others to understand what I was saying. As I am multilingual, things began to change in the language I use most frequently, Croatian. My parents started to have difficulty understanding me. I started speaking English and it was a bit better: people could understand me.

This is because Croatian is more complex. It has more sounds than English. Try pronouncing words with letters *ć, č, š, ž, đ, dž*!

But over time, English started to become a challenge like Croatian. People could not understand me. I scheduled an appointment with my GP and he sent me for an MRI to see what was going on. The scan showed that the blood vessels in my neck had narrowed due to excessive radiation from the Gamma Knife. Consequently, there was not enough blood flowing between my head and the rest of my body. The lack of oxygen caused numerous issues – headaches, asthma, not being able to exercise due to these issues. According to my GP, the narrowing of the blood vessels affected my vocal cords. He did explain how, but I forgot the technicalities. My GP did not speak of the possibilities of widening the blood vessels and I was reluctant to ask because of the possibility of more surgery, which was out of the question. I was too afraid. He did not say anything about any hazard or danger this narrowing may cause in the future but did talk about the issues that will occur – all of them are described further in this chapter. His words gave me some sort of comfort. I would definitely consider surgery if it were a 'must-do' thing. But if not, why would I put myself through such pain? Still this was a difficult package I received. At least we had found out what the problem was.

Our next step was to find a good speech therapist. The same day, we went to the Fiona Stanley Hospital in Perth to look for one. Eventually, a miraculous Russian lady started working with me. Words are not enough to explain what she did. I had appointments twice weekly for one hour, sometimes more. She made an action plan for me. Our goal was to achieve understandable speech seventy per cent of the time. Once I got to that point, I could practise on my own to gain that leftover thirty per cent. In six weeks, we achieved that goal. Very quick! Judging by the state my speech was in, I thought it would take at least five months or more. She is a true miracle worker! I am aware that it was mostly my work, but without her knowledge and guidance, the goal would not have been accomplished. That was a brisk and rapid way of solving one issue. Others persistently awaited.

My oesophagus was severely disrupted from the radiosurgery causing many other issues. The ones that affect me the most are swallowing, choking and reflux. All of that ignites asthma attacks. I am not sure which one of the three is worse. Swallowing and choking are closely related. When I swallow in the incorrect way, I start choking and then asthma ignites. The thing is that I am in the habit of eating quickly and with no water, like I did before my illness. After the illness, I had to re-learn eating the correct way, which is taking small bites, chewing them properly and drinking water to flush down the food. Half of my meals I eat with caution, but I sometimes disregard everything, and that is when problems arise. When that happens, because I do not swallow well-chewed food and I do not take small bites, I cannot swallow properly so I choke. And then, like an uninvited guest, along comes asthma. Like a domino effect, one goes down, all follow. I also choke on liquids and the process repeats itself. I am not sure what the issue is – whether it is the order of swallowing or that my swallowing is not good. Is there a proper way to swallow and has that process been lost in my case?

The last severe issue is reflux caused by stomach acid leaking up into my oesophagus. Mainly it operates in the morning or forenoon, and as usual, asthma accompanies it. The doctors say that the sphincter between my stomach and oesophagus does not work as it should. A sphincter is a circular muscle that normally maintains constriction of a natural body passage or orifice, and relaxes as required by normal physiological functioning. Mine semi-works.

I developed this new disease in 2015, and I have been battling it ever since. Aren't I blessed? Joking, but really my youth and adult years were stained and marked with unfortunate, disadvantageous and miserable events. I endured two brain tumours accompanied by different issues, physical and psychological, and now I get another disease. Nothing is easing. Things are getting worse. It is getting hard to bear all these issues.

Everything that happened makes you think *when is it going to stop? Is it ever going to stop?* I am accustomed to it but it's not easy. Nowadays in 2020, all those issues have diminished but are still present.

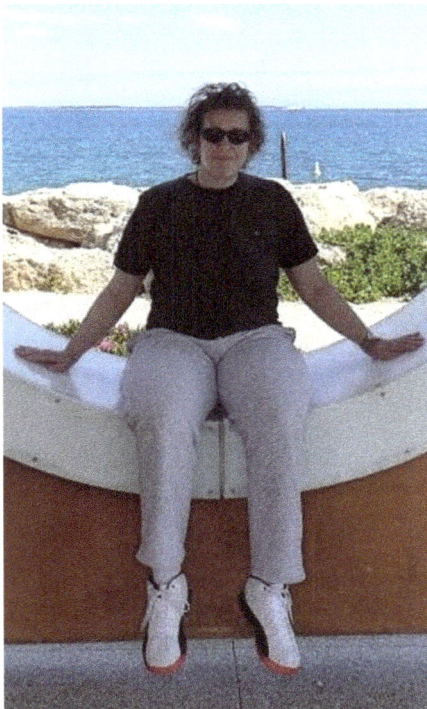

Coogee Beach, Western Australia 2020

34

Curative Remedies

◇

Never overlook the power of simplicity.

~**Robin S. Sharma**

$\mathcal{S}$ince the Gamma Knife aftermath struck hard, I needed to find something to help me cope with everything. My biggest issue, among many, was reflux. It was unbelievably bad and hard at first. It happened around eight or nine times per day, throughout the day. I did not know what to do, stomach acid mixed with food just ran out of my mouth like vomit. Horrible!

I decided to ask my GP for help. I realised that medication would not solve the problem, but I did not care. My thoughts were first to ease the exhausting problem, and search for a long-term cure later. My GP prescribed two kinds of tablets. I tried both, and neither one helped.

At that time, Mum and I were seeing a homeopathic therapist. I explained my issue and the therapist suggested using zinc tablets. She said that my problem was in the sphincter muscle.

Acid reflux occurs when the sphincter muscle at the lower end of the oesophagus relaxes at the wrong time, allowing stomach acid back up into your oesophagus. Zinc tablets help to strengthen the muscle. They would be beneficial. I followed her advice. The tablets minimised my issue, reducing my problem from eight or nine episodes a day, to one or maybe two – sometimes none. And the astonishing thing is that when I do have a bout of reflux, it does not come out of my mouth. I take one zinc tablet every day, and nowadays sometimes I forget the reflux is there. Do not misunderstand me, I still have reflux, but I have managed to get it under control with these zinc tablets.

Headaches were another daunting issue. I have coped with these since the first operation – awfully bad headaches that even painkillers did not help. They were frequent, happening ten to twelve times a month. When we came to WA, Mum started investigating possible remedies. She found that magnesium tablets can help. So, I started taking two tablets daily. The outcome was fascinating. By using them regularly, I halved the number of headaches – before magnesium I would have ten to fifteen headaches; after magnesium, only five to six headaches. I still use them regularly. Currently, I get two or three headaches a month.

Also, I discovered a hot shower helps eliminate the pain. My headaches are caused by the damage to my blood vessels caused by the radiation from the Gamma Knife surgery. The narrowed blood vessels result in less blood and therefore less oxygen flowing to my head, causing headaches. When I step under a hot shower the pain is eliminated but only when my head is under the spray. The second I cut the water, the pain comes back, but it is noticeably lower than before.

35

Physical State

◇

Take care of your body. It is the only place you have to live.

~Jim Rohn

As I mentioned before, I did not have success with physiotherapy in Croatia. The time spent in Reactiva was beneficial to some degree, but there were a lot of negatives involved. First thing was the price. It was expensive. We could have bought an apartment in Zagreb with the sum of all my sessions. Not everyone can afford to pay that kind of money based on the average pay cheque in Croatia. The second thing was Mum's job. I could not go to Zagreb alone, I needed help. Dad was in Australia and Mum was working at Gravia in Osijek, which is a three-hour drive from Zagreb. She had to take leave every two months to take me to Reactiva. Thank God her boss was understanding!

And the third thing was the fact that I was not ready for everything the Bobath therapist taught me. Like many things after the operation, it's hard to explain, but I did not entirely understand him sometimes. For example, some things Zhao, my current Bobath therapist, explains I now understand, but the same things the Bobath therapist in Reactiva explained then were not clear to me. Personally, I think I was not prepared back then for the things the Reactiva Bobath therapist told me.

In WA, I did not need to search long for the appropriate therapy, so my physiotherapy commenced fast. We arrived in September 2013, but I started to search for someone at the end of 2014. Almost immediately, I found and started working with an organisation that offers different kinds of therapy to people with disabilities. I got an occupational therapist, a speech therapist, a physiotherapist, and a support worker. I say this because in Croatia we struggled to find an appropriate physiotherapist, someone who would meet all my needs. As I exercised more intensely with my physiotherapist Zhao, I got more confident and strong enough to start walking with a frame. Currently, I can walk one or two kilometres with the frame. I cannot walk independently yet. I am able to take a few steps without help, but someone needs to be with me – just being aside.

I do not require a speech therapist or work therapy anymore. I did work with a speech therapist after the speech therapist at the Fiona Stanley Hospital. The sessions were ongoing for nearly two years, on and off. I have been told to talk as much as I can and report any difficulties. Work or occupational therapy had been stopped while I was in Croatia, and I never did it in WA. There's no need when I can do it myself at home with puzzles, models and craft – basically, anything that requires precise and specific movements.

Until now, my life has not worked out the way I planned. A lot of things happened. Bad stuff has been accompanied by even worse stuff. But I choose to continue battling everything that confronts me. I go by the saying, 'Get busy living or get busy dying!'

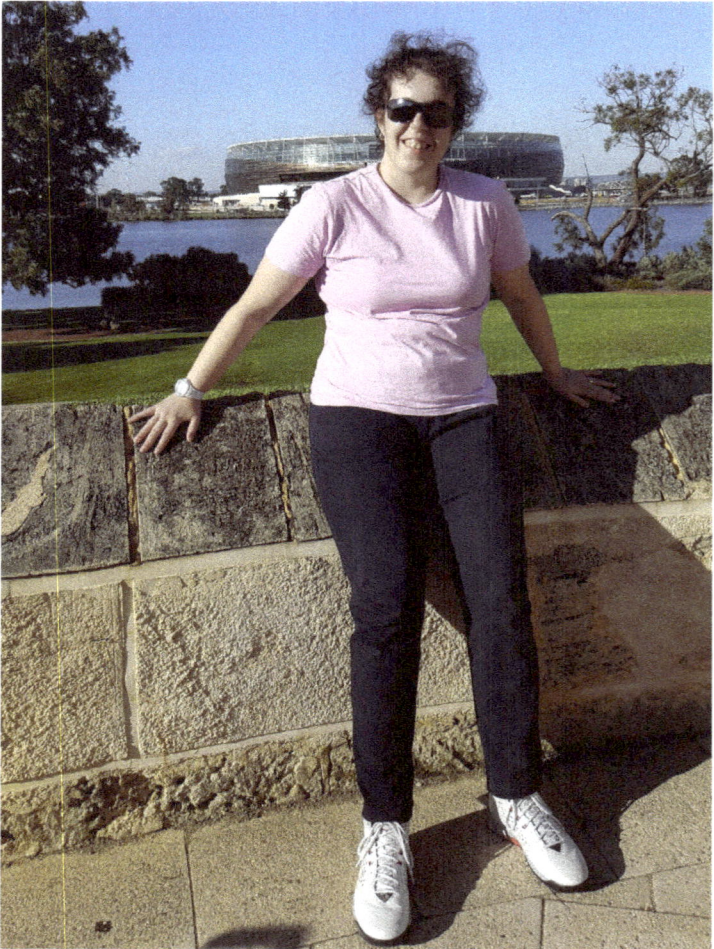

Optus stadium

36

Positively Battling Negativity

◇

*The secret of change is to focus all your energy, not on
fighting the old, but on building the new.*

~**Dan Millman**

A lot has happened since I was first diagnosed in 2003, and a lot has changed. I could not claim one hundred per cent that everything changed for the worse. I guess some changes needed to happen in order to continue a healthy lifestyle. Some changes were good, some bad, some even worse. And some were insightful. The changes are entwined in my mind, which includes my thoughts and beliefs; my soul, which includes my feelings and emotions; and lastly, my body, which includes diet and exercise. These three things – mind, body and soul – are so intertwined that it is amazing. The mind, body and soul must change accordingly and in synchronisation with each other to maintain a healthy life. Good health in mind, body and soul equals a good state of being.

For sure, the old Tihana died after the second tumour. The old me had a hard time accepting that my mind, body and soul had to be in cohesion. I am stressing those three things because I genuinely believe they must be coordinated to enable a happy and joyful life. My state before the first operation was pure chaos. I fed my body a totally unhealthy diet – loads of junk food and sugary drinks, accompanied with no exercise. My mind whirled with negative and destructive thoughts, mixed with a lot of anger and resentment, topped off with bad beliefs. My soul struggled with bad feelings, and even worse and worrying emotions. With all of that combined, one has a valid recipe for disaster. I do not know what caused the tumour and I am not implying anything, but I passionately believe that the chaos did not help.

The change was challenging. I have been deprived of my youth. My life was drastically reshaped, redesigned against my will. The first tumour impacted my life, but I managed to bounce back. Yes, there was the recovery and rehabilitation to deal with, but I still had a goal in life. A young woman's hopes and wishes were still alive. I aspired towards university, a career, relationships – a normal path in life.

Unfortunately, the second tumour destroyed everything. Now I do not know where to turn or what to do. The only thing I do know is that I need to continue with my rehabilitation. Without that, I am blank. I am positive and tend to have a different approach to life, but I still do not know what to do, or what my path will be. I've found that being positive helps. It soothes the soul.

On the one hand, my path has been very educational, but on the other, it has been hard and troublesome. I am truly thankful for all the knowledge I have gained and everything I have learnt. All that happened is thankfully in the past, but the aftermath is in the present and very visible in my life. Brain cancer transformed me into a totally different person – someone I am partly happy with, but a person still unable to let go of the past. Everything is well, but dark shadows of the past keep on haunting me and I cannot escape from them.

My motor abilities suffered more than my cognitive abilities. I am still sane. Yes, of course I would like to move and do sports like I used to, but I would not like to have endured cognitive effects. That would be even more challenging and hard to bear. Nonetheless, there are people who perceive me as a person with mental disabilities. Apart from leaving a significant trace on my motor skills and walking, what happened damaged my ability to communicate too, but not to the point of others understanding me. I speak slowly now, and some words are difficult to say. Because of that and the fact that I am in a wheelchair, most people assume that I am mentally challenged. It all seems okay, but you know those situations in which people say 'I'll check with your parents just in case'. Just in case of what? I would much prefer it if someone would flat out say 'Listen, I don't want to hurt your feelings, but I think you're challenged, so therefore you cannot be perceived as an accountable person'. At least then I would know exactly where I stand and what I can do. It hurts when people treat me as incompetent or act as if I'm not there. Incompetency and unimportance have become a reality. Not always, now that time has passed, but even now it is still present. *Sad!*

For better or worse, life does not offer the opportunity to stop and have a break to compose yourself. It unmercifully continues without even a single glance at what is left behind. Maybe that is the way it should be. Maybe life does not let us stop for our own good. Could it be possible that life is trying to tell us to keep moving, or else you will fall into the hole called depression? If we do fall, we are exposing ourselves to even greater dangers – addictions, not knowing how to pull ourselves out of that hole. Life will be even worse.

So far, my life has been full of ups and downs. It continues to be that way, but thankfully, the challenges are less great than they used to be. I choose to be positive and welcome the challenges I battle with every day. I must admit, there are days when I feel down. I am tired, frustrated, not wanting to fight anymore. But then something speaks to me, perhaps God or the universe, telling me that I should move on. And I do just that. I am aware of everything that has happened and all the repercussions it has left. Apart from the main gift I received from the tumours – ataxia and the inability to walk – other things have been affected too. Some are my sight, my hearing, uncontrolled salivation, speech issues, swallowing issues, reflux, painful headaches. Many apologies to those I left out.

Despite all that, I firmly choose to continue to fight to make the best of my life. I am happy for this third chance I have been given, and I intend to pursue it and exploit it to the end. The cancer has done the damage and there is no turning back. I cannot do anything to change what has happened. That is in the past. The only thing I can do is embrace it and continue living. When I do fall into depressing, trapped thoughts, I force myself to get up and fight. I look forward to the things that await.

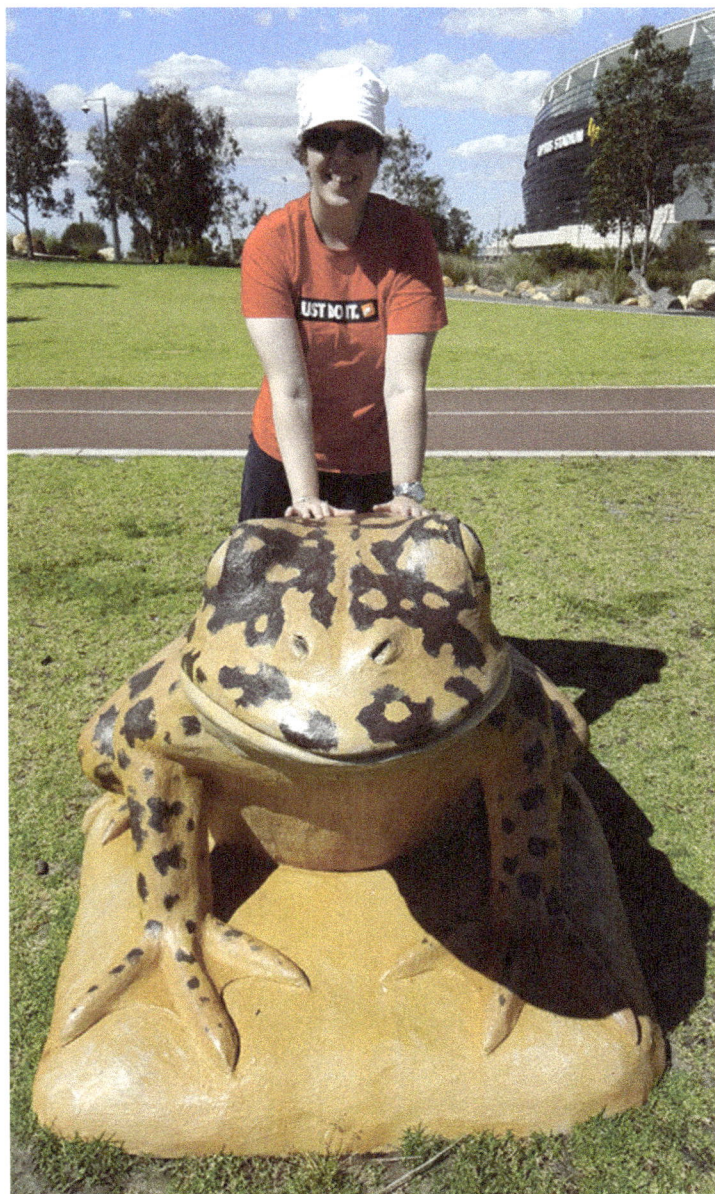

The Princess and the Frog

Epilogue

◇

Forgiveness does not change the reality of the past, but it does have the power to change your memory of the past.

~Unknown

The confronting truth is that the die has been cast. There is no going back. You can choose to play the cards you are dealt or leave them and wither until you die. I choose to fight and give it my best. In my journey to surpass brain cancer, I have used many tools such as affirmations, visualization, ETF technic[21], meditation, gratitude, religion and forgiveness. Some were helpful, some were not.

Gratitude was and is the most useful. Being grateful for what you have in the moment shifts your focus away from the things you have lost or the things you do not have. It makes you value the things you have, and it does not leave time for crying over your own destiny. People, destiny, God, the universe – forgive

---

[21] Emotional freedom technique (EFT) is an alternative treatment for physical pain and emotional distress. It is also referred to as tapping or psychological acupressure.

whomever you must in order to set yourself free. The other party is irrelevant. You gain all the benefits from the act of forgiveness. I still have a lot of forgiving to do but I have realised so far that it has brought me nothing but good. I have read somewhere that people should forgive for the purpose of gaining peace in their lives, not because the other party deserves forgiveness.

Even after everything that happened, I must admit that I appreciate and value religion. Do not get me wrong – not religion in the strict meaning of the word. It is more a casual relationship between God and me. I am not afraid of Him nor do I believe in punishment like all religions assert. Rather, I believe God is my friend, my companion, my hope, my go-to, a helping hand, my last resort. Yes, I must admit our relationship has not always been great. In my teenage years, I did not even think of religion or God. It just did not interest me. After the first operation, all the way until after the second, I blamed and cursed Him. He did this to me. I was fine until He chose to change that! Now, I do not think this was His doing. I do not know who is responsible for misfortunes and tragedies in life, but I am sure it is not Him. I am more prone to thinking that we write our own destinies. Like the proverb goes: you reap what you sow. I am a strong believer in the so-called boomerang effect or karma – if you do good, you will get good back; if you do bad, you will get bad back.

Please do not think that everything is rosy in my life. I still have a whole lot of issues to overcome. There are still negative feelings, bad emotions. A semi-trailer would not be big enough to fit it all in.

Nevertheless, I choose to go on and hope for the best.

"Forgiveness doesn't change the reality of the past, but it does have the power to change your memory of the past."

— **Paul Boese**

About the Author

◇

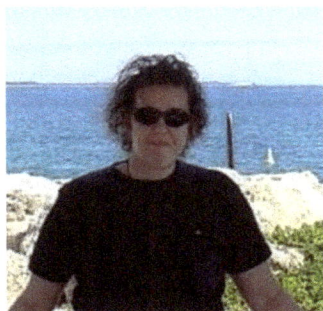

Tihana was born in Osijek, Croatia in 1984. Life was going smoothly until the age of eighteen when she was diagnosed with a brain tumour – cancer. This unfortunate event drastically changed and stigmatised her life, but some positive outcomes followed.

A year later, she enrolled in university. That proved to be a very smart move, because it not only provided knowledge, it released Tihana from the dreadful health cycle she was in and gave her a vision of a new, better future. Sadly, six years later, Tihana had a recurrence of her brain cancer, and her hopes and dreams were once again shattered. This time around, her stance on life turned to a positive and healthy approach.

From being faced with death twice, Tihana written this book to assure people that fighting and a positive approach is a winning combination.

Bibliography

Affirmation Angel. *The Power Of Your Words: Lighthearted Inspiration From An Angel's Point Of View*. Brolga Publishing; Melbourne, 2013.

Anić, Vladimir and Goldštain, Ivo. *Rječnik Stranih Riječi*. Novi Liber; Zagreb, 1999.

Byrne, Rhonda. *The Magic*. Simon & Schuster; Sydney, 2012.

Canfield, Jack, Hansen, Mark Victor and Newmark, Amy. *Chicken Soup For The Soul: From Lemons To Lemonade*. Chicken Soup for the Soul Publishing; 2013.

Canfield, Jack, Hansen, Mark Victor, Gabellini, Jeanna and Gregory, Eva. *Life Lessons For Mastering The Law Of Attraction*. Florida, 2004.

Chan, Melanie. *Life Coaching – Life Changing: How To Use The Law Of Attraction To Make Positive Changes In Your Life*. O–Books; Washington, 2012.

Dispenza, Dr Joe. *Breaking The Habit Of Being Yourself: How To Lose Your Mind And Create A New One*. Hay House; California, 2012.

Dispenza, Dr Joe. *You Are The Placebo: Making Your Mind Matter.* Hay House; Australia, 2018.

Hicks, Esther and Jerry*; Ask And It Is Given: Learning To Manifest The Law Of Attraction.* Hay House; Sydney, 2015.

Matthews, Andrew. *Slijedi Svoje Srce.* Stanek d.o.o.; Varaždin, 2001.

Miljković, Dubravka and Rijavec, Majda. *Razgovori Sa Zrcalom.* IEP d.o.o.; Zagreb, 2001.

Murphy, Dr Joseph. *Moč Vaše Podsvjest.* V.B.Z. d.o.o.; Zagreb, 2001.

Newmark, Amy and Anderson, Antony. *Chicken Soup For The Soul: The Power Of Forgiveness.* Chicken Soup for the Soul Publishing; 2014.

Prather, Hugh. *The Little Book Of Letting Go.* Conari Press; Newburyport, 2000.

Tibbits, Dr Dick and Halliday, Steve. *Forgive To Live: How Forgiveness Can Save Your Life.* Florida, 2006.

Walsch, Neale Donald. *Conversations With God, Books 1–3.* Hodder & Stoughton; London, 1997.